Fundamentals of Clinical Psychopharmacology

Fundamentals of Clinical Psychopharmacology

Second edition

Edited by

Ian M Anderson MD FRCPsych
Senior Lecturer in Psychiatry
University of Manchester
Manchester, UK

Ian C Reid PhD MRCPsych
Professor of Psychiatry
Medical School
Foresterhill, Aberdeen, UK

Provided as a service
to medicine by
Wyeth

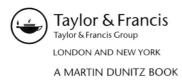

Taylor & Francis
Taylor & Francis Group

LONDON AND NEW YORK

A MARTIN DUNITZ BOOK

© 2002, 2004 British Association for Psychopharmacology

First published in the United Kingdom in 2002
by Taylor & Francis, an imprint of the Taylor & Francis Group, 2 Park Square, Milton
Park, Abingdon, Oxfordshire, OX14 4RN

Tel.:   +44 (0) 1235 828 600
Fax.:   +44 (0) 1235 829 000
E-mail: info@dunitz.co.uk
Website: http://www.dunitz.co.uk

Second edition 2004

Although every effort has been made to ensure that all owners of copyright material have
been acknowledged in this publication, we would be glad to acknowledge in subsequent
reprints or editions any omissions brought to our attention.

Although every effort has been made to ensure that drug doses and other information
are presented accurately in this publication, the ultimate responsibility rests with the
prescribing physician. Neither the publishers nor the authors can be held responsible for
errors or for any consequences arising from the use of information contained herein. For
detailed prescribing information or instructions on the use of any product or procedure
discussed herein, please consult the prescribing information or instructional material
issued by the manufacturer.

A CIP record for this book is available from the British Library.

Library of Congress Cataloging-in-Publication Data

Data available on application

ISBN 1-84184-521-3

Printed and bound in Great Britain by The Cromwell Press ltd, Trowbridge, Wilts.

Contents

Contributors   vii

Preface to the Second Edition   ix

A note on BANs and rINNs   xii

List of abbreviations   xiii

1 Neuropharmacology and drug action   1
   Charles A Marsden

2 Pharmacokinetics and pharmacodynamics   27
   Ian Anderson

3 Antipsychotics   41
   Michael Travis and Ian C Reid

4 Antidepressants and electroconvulsive therapy   59
   Ian C Reid

5 'Mood stabilisers': lithium and anticonvulsants   79
   Allan Young and Ian C Reid

6 Anxiolytics   95
   Stephen J Cooper

7 Drugs of abuse   109
   Anne Lingford-Hughes

8 Drug treatments for child and adolescent disorders 123
   David Coghill

9 Drugs for dementia   135
   N Harry P Allen

10 Clinical trial methodology   145
   Stephen M Lawrie and R Hamish McAllister-Williams

Index   163

Contributors

N Harry P Allen
Consultant Old Age Psychiatrist
York House
Manchester Royal Infirmary
Oxford Road
Manchester M13 9WL, UK

Ian M Anderson
Senior Lecturer in Psychiatry
Neuroscience and Psychiatry Unit
University of Manchester
Room G809
Stopford Building
Oxford Road
Manchester M13 7PT, UK

David Coghill
Senior Lecturer and Honorary
    Consultant in Child and
    Adolescent Psychiatry
Centre for Child Health
19 Dudhope Terrace
Dundee DD3 6HH, UK

Stephen J Cooper
Senior Lecturer in Psychiatry
Department of Mental Health
Queen's University Belfast
Whitla Medical Building
97 Lisburn Road
Belfast BT9 7BL, UK

Stephen M Lawrie
Senior Clinical Research Fellow
Kennedy Tower
Royal Edinburgh Hospital
Edinburgh EH10 5HF, UK

Anne Lingford-Hughes
Senior Lecturer in Biological
    Psychiatry and Addiction
Division of Psychiatry
University of Bristol
Cotham House, Cotham Hill
Bristol BS6 6JL, UK

R Hamish McAllister-Williams
Senior Lecturer and Honorary
    Consultant Psychiatrist
School of Neurology
    Neurobiology and Psychiatry
University of Newcastle upon Tyne
Department of Psychiatry
Leazes Wing
Royal Victoria Infirmary
Newcastle upon Tyne NE1 4LP, UK

Charles A Marsden
Professor of Neuropharmacology
School of Biomedical Sciences
Institute of Neuroscience
University of Nottingham Medical
    School
Queen's Medical Centre
Nottingham NG7 2UH, UK

Ian C Reid
Professor of Psychiatry
IMS Building
Medical School
Foresterhill
Aberdeen AB25 2ZD, UK

Michael Travis
Consultant Psychiatrist and
    Honorary Senior Lecturer
Section of Clinical
    Neuropharmacology P051
Division of Psychological Medicine
Institute of Psychiatry
De Crespigny Park
London SE5 8AF, UK

Allan Young
Professor in General Psychiatry
Department of Psychiatry
Royal Victoria Infirmary
Queen Victoria Road
Newcastle upon Tyne NE1 4LP, UK

Preface to the Second Edition

The first edition of *Fundamentals of Clinical Psychopharmacology* was only published in 2002 but the aim of the book has always been to provide more up-to-date information than is usually available in textbooks. The field of psychopharmacology is moving rapidly and unfortunately for the contributors (and editors) this has meant having to update the information after a fairly short interval. We are grateful to everyone for their enthusiasm and hard work and also to the publishers for being able and willing to respond flexibly and quickly. This means that hopefully the information will still be 'in-date' by publication.

For this new edition we have updated all the chapters and included a new one on the controversial topic of drugs for child and adolescent psychiatric disorders. It has been an opportunity to correct any mistakes that had crept into the first edition, and we have continued to put drug prescribing into the context of UK guidance and regulation. Given the trend for more regulation and central control over the use of drugs, we believe it is important for those involved in prescribing to be aware of this (whatever their views about it!).

This book has developed from the acclaimed twice-yearly British Association for Psychopharmacology (BAP) 'Psychopharmacology Course for Psychiatrists in Training'. It resulted from requests from the trainees to complement the course, and the chapters in the book reflect, and extend, the course content, ranging from basic neuroscience to the analysis of clinical trials. It is not a comprehensive textbook of psychopharmacology but provides what we believe to be the core of clinically relevant information about drugs in the context of current knowledge about the biological basis of the disorders which they treat. There is a UK focus in aspects of prescribing practice but the science and clinical information are international.

We hope that the book will be of particular value to trainees sitting the membership examinations of The Royal College of Psychiatrists in the UK, but it should also be useful to other clinicians, scientists and students who seek concise and up-to-date information about current psychopharmacological knowledge and practice.

The contributors are leading UK psychopharmacologists who have presented the course. However, as the course has evolved over the years there are many others who have been involved in developing the material and they are acknowledged below.

Just a brief note about the BAP. It was founded in 1974, with the general intention of bringing together those from clinical and experimental disciplines as well as members of the pharmaceutical industry involved in the study of psychopharmacology. The BAP arranges scientific meetings, fosters research and teaching, encourages the publication of research, produces clinical guidelines, publishes the *Journal of Psychopharmacology* and provides guidance and information to the public on matters relevant to psychopharmacology. The publication of the second edition of *Fundamentals of Clinical Psychopharmacology* continues its educational tradition. Membership of the BAP is open to anyone with a relevant degree related to neuroscience including clinical, medical, nursing or pharmacy degrees. If you are reading this book, you are probably eligible to join and we would strongly encourage you to consider doing so. You can find out more on our website (http://www.bap.org.uk) or contact us at:

British Association for Psychopharmacology
36 Cambridge Place
Hills Road
Cambridge CB2 1NS
UK

Ian M Anderson
Ian C Reid

Acknowledgements

We would like to thank the following colleagues who have been involved in the development of the course material:

Dr Clive Adams
Dr David Baldwin
Dr David Balfour
Prof. Thomas Barnes
Dr Geoff Bennett
Prof. Philip Cowen
Dr Mark Daglish
Prof. Bill Deakin
Dr Colin Dourish
Prof. Barry Everitt
Professor Nicol Ferrier
Dr Sophia Frangou
Dr Sasha Gartside
Prof. Guy Goodwin
Dr John Hughes
Dr Eileen Joyce
Prof. Robert Kerwin
Prof. David King
Dr Andrea Malizia
Prof. David Nutt
Dr Veronica O'Keane
Dr Carmine Pariante
Dr Lyn Pilowsky
Dr Clare Stanford
Dr Stuart Watson

A note on BANs and rINNS

Until now we have been able in the UK to use our well-established national naming system, British Approved Names (BANs), to identify drugs. However, in order to avoid confusion (and to meet requirements in both European and UK legislation), we are now instructed to use recommended International Non-Proprietary Names (rINNs). This is co-ordinated by the World Health Organization (but to British eyes looks like a further step in the Americanisation of UK English). The name changes are mostly (but not all) minor, but it is with a heavy heart we see the loss of 'ph' to be replaced by 'f' in words like 'amphetamine'. A minor reprieve is the saving of adrenaline and noradrenaline, which will at least allow us some continuing dignity.

The changes became effective on 1 December 2003 with industry having between one and two years (depending whether the name is of the active substance) to finalise the name changes. In practice, prescribers are advised to familiarise themselves with the name changes, prescribe and dispense using only rINNs by 30 June 2004 and to inform patients when the names of the medicines on their prescription and dispensed medicine change. Further information is available from:

http://medicines.mhra.gov.uk/inforesources/productinfo/banrinn.htm.

While it is likely that the old names will take time to die out, especially away from the clinical setting, we have used rINNs throughout this book but have given both names where there might be confusion (e.g. dosulepin/ dothiepin, trihexphenidyl/benzhexol).

List of abbreviations

1-PP	1-pyramidyl piperazine
5-HT	5-hydroxytryptamine, serotonin
5-HIAA	5-hydroxyindoleacetic acid
AC	adenylate cyclase
ACE	angiotensin-converting enzyme
ACh	acetylcholine
AD	Alzheimer's disease
ADAS	Alzheimer's Disease Assessment Scale
ADHD	attention deficit/hyperactivity disorder
ADL	activities of daily living
ALDH	aldehyde dehydrogenase
AMP	adenosine monophosphate
AMPA	amino-3-hydroxy-5-methyl-isoxazole propionate
AMTS	Abbreviated Mental Test Score
AP5	2-amino-5-phosphopentanoic acid
APP	amyloid precursor protein
ATP	adenosine triphosphate
AUC	area under the curve
β-CCE	ethyl-β-carboline-3-carboxylate
BD	bipolar disorder
BDZ	benzodiazepine
BNF	British National Formulary
BPSD	behavioural and psychiatric symptoms of dementia
CA	cannabinoid
Ca^{2+}	calcium
cAMP	cyclic adenosine monophosphate, cyclic AMP
CBT	cognitive behavioural therapy
CCK	cholecystokinin
CDR	Clinical Dementia Rating

CIBIC	Clinicians Interview Based Impression of Change
Cl⁻	chloride
C_{max}	maximum plasma concentration (pharmacokinetics)
CNS	central nervous system
CO_2	carbon dioxide
COMT	catechol-*O*-methyltransferase
C_p	plasma concentration (pharmacokinetics)
CRF	corticotrophin-releasing factor
CSF	cerebrospinal fluid
CYP450	cytochrome P450
D	dopamine (used for receptor terminology)
DA	dopamine
DAG	diacylglycerol
DOPAC	dihydroxyphenylacetic acid
DSM-IV	Fourth revision of the Diagnostic and Statistical Manual of Mental Disease (American Psychiatric Association)
ECG	electrocardiogram
ECS	electroconvulsive shock (animals)
ECT	electroconvulsive therapy
EPSE	extrapyramidal side-effects
GABA	γ-aminobutyric acid
GAD	generalised anxiety disorder
GDP	guanine diphosphate
G	guanine nucleotide
G_i	inhibitory G-protein
GTP	guanine triphosphate
G_s	stimulatory G-protein
H	histamine
HPA	hypothalmic—pituitary—adrenal
HRT	hormone replacement therapy
IADL	Instrumental Activities of Daily Living
ICD-10	Tenth revision of the International Classification of Diseases (World Health Organization)
IDDD	Interview for Deterioration in Daily Living in Dementia
IP_3	inositol trisphosphate
IPT	interpersonal therapy
ITT	intention-to-treat
K⁺	potassium
LAAM	levo-alpha-acetylmethadol

LC	locus coeruleus
LOCF	last observation carried forward
LSD	lysergic acid diethylamide
LTP	long-term potentiation
M	muscarinic
MAO	monoamine oxidase
MAOI	monoamine oxidase inhibitor
MDA	methylenedioxyamphetamine
MDD	major depressive disorder
MDEA	methylenedioxyethylamphetamine
MDMA	methylenedioxymethamphetamine
Mg^{2+}	magnesium
MHRA	Medicines and Healthcare products Regulatory Authority (UK)
MK-801	dizocilpine
MMRM	mixed effects model repeated measures
MMSE	Mini-Mental State Examination
MOUSEPAD	Manchester and Oxford Universities Scale for the Psychopathological Assessment of Dementia
NA	noradrenaline
Na^+	sodium
NARI	noradrenaline re-uptake inhibitor
NaSSa	noradrenaline- and serotonin-specific antidepressant
NICE	National Institute for Clinical Excellence (UK)
NK	neurokinin
NMDA	*N*-methyl D-aspartate
NMS	neuroleptic malignant syndrome
NPI	Neuropsychiatric Inventory
NPY	neuropeptide Y
NSAID	nonsteroidal anti-inflammatory drug
NT	neurotensin
OCD	obsessive—compulsive disorder
PAG	periaqueductal grey
PCP	phencyclidine
PEM	prescription event monitoring
PET	positron emission tomography
PTSD	post-traumatic stress disorder
Q	quantity of drug (pharmacokinetics)
QTc	interval between Q and T waves on the electrocardiogram corrected for heart rate
RCT	randomised controlled trial

SNRI	serotonin and noradrenaline re-uptake inhibitor
SPECT	single photon emission computerised tomography
SSRI	selective serotonin re-uptake inhibitor
$t_{1/2}$	half-life (pharmacokinetics)
TCAs	tricyclic antidepressants
THA	tacrine, tetrahydroaminoacridine
THC	tetrahydrocannabinol
t_{max}	time to maximum (peak) plasma concentration
TRH	thyrotropin-releasing hormone
V_d	volume of distribution (pharmacokinetics)
VTA	ventral tegmental area
Z^{2+}	zinc

1 Neuropharmacology and drug action

Introduction

This chapter will concentrate on the mechanisms by which drugs alter neuro-transmission of relevance to the treatment of psychiatric disorders.

■ The major site of action for drugs used in psychiatry is the synapse and in particular those utilising amines or amino acids as neurotransmitters.
■ The majority of the drugs act either presynaptically to influence levels of the neurotransmitter in the synaptic cleft, or by altering the functional state of the postsynaptic receptors.

Neurotransmission

Neurotransmission describes the process by which information is transferred from one neurone to another across the synapse (Fig. 1.1). It involves:

■ the release of a neurotransmitter from the presynaptic nerve ending in response to the arrival of an action potential and influx of calcium (Ca^{2+});
■ the subsequent activation of a receptor on the membrane of the post-synaptic neurone.

Activation of the postsynaptic receptor may result either in:

■ excitation – membrane depolarisation; or
■ inhibition – membrane hyperpolarisation.

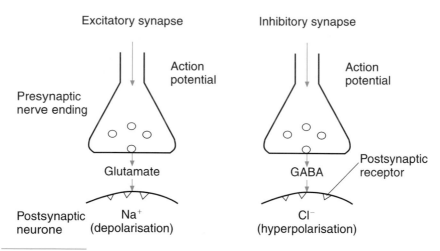

Figure 1.1 *Synaptic transmission involves the release of a neurotransmitter from the presynaptic nerve ending and its binding to a postsynaptic receptor to produce a change in function (excitation or inhibition) in the postsynaptic neurone.*

These may be due to either:

- a direct effect on an ion channel (fast neurotransmission; Fig. 1.2); or
- enzyme inhibition via a guanine nucleotide binding (G) protein-coupled second-messenger system (slow neurotransmission; Fig. 1.2) (see receptor mechanisms below).

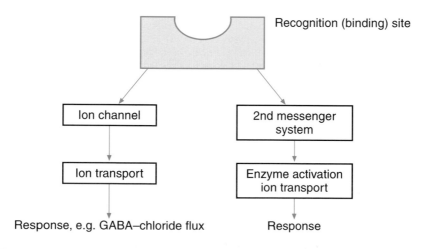

Figure 1.2 *Fast-acting transmitters act by opening an ion channel (e.g. glutamate and GABA) while slower-acting neurotransmitters, often involved in tonic regulation, act through G-protein-coupled receptors (e.g. amines such as DA and 5-HT).*

The initial receptor response (i.e. excitation or inhibition) does not necessarily describe the final functional output, for example inhibition of an inhibitory neurone will cause disinhibition of the next neurone in the chain and thus a net excitatory response. Figure 1.3 shows an important example of disinhibition.

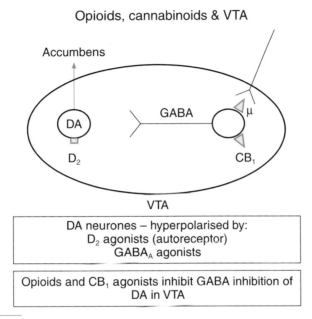

Opioids, cannabinoids & VTA

DA neurones – hyperpolarised by:
D_2 agonists (autoreceptor)
$GABA_A$ agonists

Opioids and CB_1 agonists inhibit GABA inhibition of DA in VTA

Figure 1.3 *An example of disinhibition. DA neurones in the ventral tegmental area (VTA) project to the mesolimbic areas. GABA neurones in the VTA inhibit DA neuronal firing. Opioids (e.g. metencephalin) released in the VTA stimulate opioid µ receptors causing inhibition of the GABA neurones resulting in disinhibition (activation) of the DA neurones and increased release of DA in the nucleus accumbens. Cannabinoid (CB) agonists (e.g. tetrahydrocannabinol, THC) also disinhibit this pathway through the activation of CB_1 receptors located on GABA neurones. This effect is related to the dependence liability of opioid drugs.*

Behaviour is thus the result of a complex interplay between many neurones and it is very difficult therefore to explain a particular behaviour as being the result of the action of a single neurotransmitter.

Co-existence of neurotransmitters

■ The original concept of chemical neurotransmission stated that only one active substance (neurotransmitter) was released presynaptically.

■ This has been modified to incorporate the idea of coexistence when two or more biologically active substances are released in response to an action potential.

- However, all the substances released do not necessarily act as neurotransmitters (i.e. produce a functional response in the postsynaptic neurone).
- Some substances released from nerve endings act as neuromodulators (i.e. interact with the neurotransmitter to either facilitate or reduce its action without causing functional effects of their own).
- Amines – dopamine (DA), noradrenaline (NA, also called norepinephrine), 5-hydroxytryptamine (5-HT, also called serotonin) and acetylcholine (ACh) – commonly co-exist with various neuropeptides, e.g. cholecystokinin (CCK), neurotensin (NT) and thyrotrophin-releasing hormone (TRH); which act as either
  - full neurotransmitters (i.e. produce a functional response on their own); or
  - as neuromodulators (when they modulate the responsiveness of the amine neurotransmitter).
- Coexistence is probably the normal state of affairs though there is little detailed understanding of its functional importance or about the ways it could impact on drug treatment.

Neurotransmitters

In addition to the major neurotransmitters implicated in psychiatric disorders and targets for drugs (DA, NA, 5-HT, ACh, GABA and glutamate), Table 1.1 also lists some of the other neurotransmitters/neuromodulators and in particular some of the numerous neuropeptides found in the brain.

- There are over 60 neuropeptides identified; the best understood are the encephalins which activate opioid receptors.
- There is interest in the neurokinins (substance P, neurokinin A and neurokinin B) and their receptors (NK_1, NK_2 and NK_3) as possible targets for antidepressant and antipsychotic drugs.
- Neurotensin (NT) had been postulated as a possible antischizophrenic target because of evidence for coexistence with DA and modulation of DA-induced behaviours.
- CCK administration can induce panic attacks (especially in panic disorder patients); the mechanisms are not fully understood but may include both brain and peripheral mechanisms. However CCK receptor antagonists have not been successful antipanic drugs but this may in part relate to poor brain penetration of the compounds.

Table 1.1 *Central nervous system neurotransmitters and neuromodulators*

The main neurotransmitters and neuromodulators and a few neuropeptides and the main disorders with which they are associated

Substance	Disorder
Amines	
Acetylcholine (ACh)	Alzheimer's disease
Dopamine (DA)	Parkinson's disease, schizophrenia
Noradrenaline (NA)	Anxiety, depression, cognition, schizophrenia, hypertension
Adrenaline	Hypertension
5-Hydroxytryptamine (serotonin, 5-HT)	Depression, anxiety/panic/OCD, schizophrenia, Alzheimer's disease, migraine, hallucinations, feeding disorders
Histamine (H)	Arousal, cognition
Amino acids	
Glutamate	Neurodegeneration
γ-Aminobutyric acid (GABA)	Anxiety, Huntington's disease, epilepsy
Peptides	
Met/Leu-Enkephalin	Pain, mood
β-Endorphin	Pain, mood
Substance P/tachykinins	Huntington's disease, depression
Vasopressin	Cognition, hypertension
Cholecystokinin (CCK)	Anxiety, pain
Neurotensin (NT)	Schizophrenia
Thyrotrophin-releasing hormone (TRH)	Arousal, motor neurone disease
Neuropeptide Y (NPY)	Feeding disorders, blood pressure
Corticotrophin-releasing factor (CRF)	Anxiety, depression
Orexins	Circadian function disorders, feeding disorders, response to stress
Other	
Endocannabinoids (e.g. anandamide)	Pain, schizophrenia, feeding disorders

■ Given the role of the hypothalamic–pituitary–adrenal (HPA) axis in depression, corticotrophin-releasing factor (CRF) receptors (CRF_1, CRF_2) antagonists are currently under clinical evaluation as antidepressants.

■ Orexins A and B (hypocretins) are closely related neuropeptides derived from a single gene. They act on OX_1 and OX_2 receptors which are highly expressed in the lateral hypothalamus and other brain areas involved in stress regulation. Orexins were initially identified as important regulators of feeding but are now seen as involved in circadian function, sleep and response to stress including neuroendocrine control.

■ Other potential targets for drugs:

– The endocannabinoid system in the brain; annandamide is one of several endogenous agonists of cannabinoid type 1 (CB_1) and type 2 (CB_2) receptors. CB_1 receptors are found in the brain and are potential targets for the treatment of pain and various mood disorders. CB_2 receptors are associated with the immune system.

– Neurosteroids (i.e. steroids either made within the brain or with access to the brain). These interact with steroid receptors and modulate the function of $GABA_A$ receptor function and are thus potential anti-anxiety drug targets (see Chapter 6).

– Various neurotrophic factors also have an important role not only in the normal development of the brain but they also act to maintain synaptic function, and in some cases regulation of transmitter release, in the adult brain. An example is brain-derived neurotrophic factor (BDNF), the expression of which is increased by chronic antidepressant treatment in animals and so may be involved in the mechanism of action of these drugs.

Organisation of transmitter pathways

The major neurotransmitter pathways – and those most important in psychopharmacology – can be divided organisationally into three groups:

■ Long ascending and descending axonal pathways derived from discrete neuronal cell groups located within specific brain nuclei. This is seen with catecholamine (DA, NA) and indolamine (5-HT) as well as many cholinergic (ACh) pathways.

■ Long and short axonal pathways derived from neuronal cell bodies widely distributed throughout the brain. These pathways are associated with the major excitatory (glutamate) and inhibitory (GABA) neurotransmitters. They lack the very precise organisational structures of the amine pathways.

■ Short intraregional pathways including interneurones within the cerebral cortex, striatum, etc. Often associated with GABA inhibition but also various neuropeptides (e.g. somatostatin in the cerebral cortex).

Receptor mechanisms

Receptors and transporters (responsible for reuptake of neurotransmitters; see below) are the main target for drug action.

Receptors for neurotransmitters are located on membranes and can be:

- directly coupled to an ion channel (also called ionotropic receptors) so concerned with fast neurotransmission (e.g. N-methyl-D-aspartate (NMDA)-type of glutamate receptor, $GABA_A$ and nicotinic types of ACh receptors); or
- coupled to an intracellular effector system via a G-protein (also called metabotropic receptors), and so responsible for slow neurotransmission (e.g. DA, NA, most 5-HT and muscarinic ACh receptors); or
- linked to other systems such as the membrane kinase-linked receptors (growth factors, insulin) and intracellular receptors that control gene transcription (steroids).

Ion channel-linked receptors

- Ion channel-linked receptors are protein structures containing about 20 transmembrane segments (i.e. they cross the cell membrane 20 times) so arranged to form a central channel.
- Binding of the transmitter to the receptor opens the channel to specific ions.
- Ion channel opening occurs in milliseconds, thus there are rapid excitatory or inhibitory effects depending on which ion the channel is permeable to.

G-protein receptors (Fig. 1.4)

- G-protein receptors are so named because their action is linked to the binding of guanyl nucleotides.
- They consist of seven transmembrane-spanning sections, one of which is larger than the rest and interacts with the G-protein.
- The G-protein has three subunits (α, β, γ) with the α unit containing guanyl triphosphatase (GTPase) activity.
- When the transmitter or agonist binds to the receptor, α-guanyl triphosphate (α-GTP) is released, which then can either activate or inhibit one of two major second messenger systems:
  - Adenylate cyclase/cyclic adenosine monophosphate (cAMP). Production of cAMP activates various protein kinases, which in turn influence the function of various enzymes, carriers, etc. Adenylate cyclase can either be stimulated (excitation) or inhibited (inhibition) (Fig. 1.4).

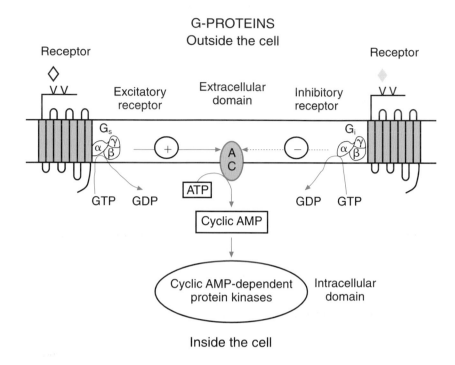

Figure 1.4 *G-proteins couple the receptor-binding site to the second messenger system and they consist of three subunits (α, β, γ) anchored to the seven transmembrane helices that form the receptor. Coupling of the α subunit to an agonist-occupied receptor causes bound guanine diphosphate (GDP) to exchange with guanine triphosphate (GTP) and the resulting α–GTP complex leaves the receptor to interact with a target protein (an enzyme such as adenylate cyclase (AC), or an ion channel). There is then hydrolysis of the bound GTP to GDP and the α subunit links again to the βγ subunit. The G-protein mechanism can be either inhibitory (G_i) or excitatory (G_s). In summary, the G-proteins provide the link between the ligand recognition site and the effector system.*

- Phospholipase C/inositol trisphosphate (IP_3)/diacylglycerol (DAG). Activation of this system results in the formation of two intracellular messengers (IP_3 and DAG). IP_3 increases free calcium (Ca^{2+}) thus activating various enzymes. DAG activates protein kinase C, which in turn regulates various cellular functions (Fig. 1.5).
■ G-proteins can also control potassium (K^+) and Ca^{2+} channel function thus regulating membrane excitability and transmitter release, e.g. 5-HT_{1A} receptor activation inhibits adenylate cyclase and increases K^+ conductance (hyperpolarisation).

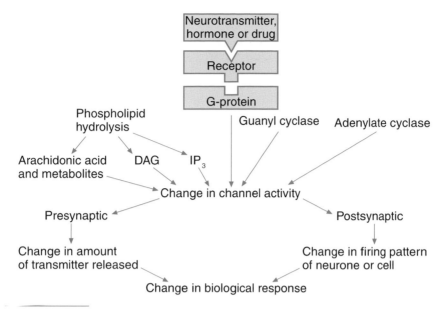

Figure 1.5 *G-protein-coupled receptors are linked to several second messenger (effector systems). The most important in psychopharmacology are the adenylate cyclase and phospholipid hydrolysis mechanisms.*

Specific examples of receptor types

■ Glutamate is an example of a fast-acting excitatory transmitter where the receptors (NMDA and AMPA) are directly linked to a sodium (Na^+) channel

■ γ-Amino butyric acid (GABA) is the major fast-acting inhibitory transmitter. Activation of the $GABA_A$ receptor, which is linked to a chloride (Cl^-) channel, results in an influx of Cl^- into the neurone causing hyperpolarisation.

■ The amine neurotransmitters (DA, NA, 5-HT and ACh):
  – generally act as slow excitatory or inhibitory transmitters depending upon their receptor coupling system (see below). This explains their wide role in the long-term modulation of behaviour;
  – however, some amine receptors are directly coupled to ion channels ($5-HT_3$, nicotinic ACh receptors).

Receptor location

■ The location of the receptor determines its effects on neurotransmission (Fig. 1.6)

■ Neurotransmitter receptors are mostly located on a membrane on the far side of the synapse to the point of release. These postsynaptic receptors may be located on:
  – dendrites or the soma of a neurone, in which case they regulate cell firing; or
  – a nerve terminal in which case the function will be to regulate neurotransmitter release; in this situation the receptor is sometimes referred to as a *presynaptic heteroceptor.*
■ Receptors located on the same type of neurone that releases the neurotransmitter that activates it are termed *autoreceptors* and are concerned with the autoregulation (normally inhibitory feedback) of neuronal firing and terminal transmitter release.
  – When the autoreceptor is located on the soma or dendrites of the neurone it is termed a *somatodendritic autoreceptor* and regulates neuronal firing.
  – When the autoreceptor is located on the terminal it is termed a *terminal autoreceptor* and regulates release.

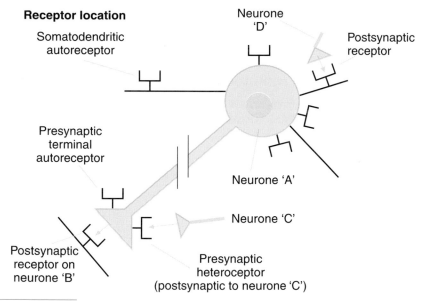

Figure 1.6 *The nomenclature used to describe receptor location on neurones. Starting with 'Neurone A', neurotransmitter released at the terminals will interact with POSTSYNAPTIC receptors on 'Neurone B'. Similarly, neurotransmitter released from 'Neurone D' will interact with postsynaptic receptor on 'Neurone A'. Neurotransmitter released from 'Neurone A' will also regulate its own release by interacting with the TERMINAL AUTORECEPTOR or affect neuronal firing by interacting with the SOMATODENDRITIC AUTORECEPTOR. Release of neurotransmitter from 'Neurone A' can also be regulated by activation of PRESYNAPTIC HETEROCEPTORS on the terminals, which are postsynaptic receptors activated by neurotransmitter from 'Neurone C'.*

– The DA autoreceptor at both sites is the D_2 receptor; similarly, the NA autoreceptor is the α_2 receptor. With 5-HT neurones the 5-HT$_{1A}$ receptor acts as the main somatodendritic autoreceptor but the 5-HT$_{1B/1D}$ receptor is the terminal autoreceptor.

Dopamine (DA)

Pathways and functions

DA-containing neuronal cell bodies are located in three discrete areas (Fig. 1.7):

■ *Substantia nigra* – axons project from this midbrain area to the basal ganglia (dorsal striatum, caudate-putamen).
   – They are involved in the initiation of motor plans and motor co-ordination.
   – This pathway is the primary site of degeneration in Parkinson's disease.
   – Antipsychotic drugs (D_2-receptor antagonists) produce motor disturbances by blocking D_2 receptors in the caudate-putamen).

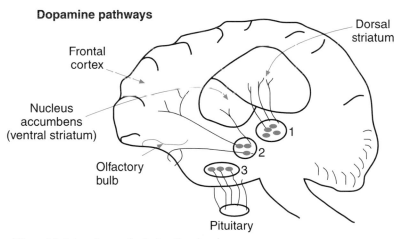

1. Nigrostriatal pathway (substantia nigra)
   Parkinson's disease, initiation of motor plans
2. Mesocortical and mesolimbic pathways (ventral tegmental area, VTA)
   Schizophrenia, reward and motivation
3. Tuberoinfundibular pathway (median eminence)
   Prolactin release

Figure 1.7 *Diagram of the main DA pathways in the brain. Note the discrete localisation of the neuronal cell bodies in the substantia nigra, VTA and median eminence.*

■ *Ventral tegmental area* (VTA) – axons project to the accumbens (ventral striatum), amygdala and prefrontal cortex.
  – These are referred to as the mesolimbic and mesocortical DA pathways.
  – These pathways are considered important in schizophrenia and an important site of action for antipsychotic drugs (D_2 and D_4 antagonists).
  – They are also strongly associated with motivation, reward behaviour and dependence produced by amfetamines (which release DA), cocaine (which blocks DA re-uptake) and opioids, cannabinoids and nicotine, all of which indirectly increase the firing of DA release in the terminal regions.

■ *Tuberoinfundibular DA pathway* – neurones in the median eminence that project to the pituitary.
  – Release of DA inhibits prolactin release via activation of D_2 receptors.
  – Drugs that antagonise D_2 receptors (e.g. antipsychotics) increase prolactin secretion causing amenorrhoea, etc.

Synthesis and metabolism

■ DA is formed by the hydroxylation of tyrosine to dihydroxyphenylanine (DOPA) by tyrosine hydroxylase followed by decarboxylation to DA by DOPA decarboxylase.
■ Following release, DA is taken back up into the presynaptic terminal by the DA transporter.
■ DA is also metabolised by mitochondrial monoamine oxidase (MAO) and by the membrane-bound catechol-O-methyltransferase (COMT) enzyme to form the endproduct homovallinic acid (HVA) (Table 1.2).
■ Both MAO and COMT inhibitors are used in the symptomatic treatment of Parkinson's disease and MAO inhibitors in depression.
■ DA release is under inhibitory autoreceptor feedback regulation by the presynaptic D_2 and/or D_3 dopamine receptor; activation of these receptors results in the inhibition of DA release (Fig. 1.8).

DA receptors

■ Five DA receptors have been identified using pharmacological and molecular biological methods.
■ These consist of two families: the 'D_1 like' with D_1 (also further subdivided into D_{1A} and D_{1B}) and D_5 receptors, which are positively coupled to cAMP; and the 'D_2 like' (D_2, D_3, D_4) which inhibit cAMP.
■ There are further variants, with short and long forms of the D_2 receptor,

Table 1.2 *Neurotransmitter synthesis and metabolism. Summary of the enzymes involved in the synthesis and metabolism of amine and amino acid neurotransmitters*

Transmitter	Precursor	Synthesis enzymes	Inactivation
Acetylcholine (ACh)	Choline	CAT	Enzymatic (AChE)
	Acetyl Co-A		Choline recycled
Dopamine (DA)	Tyrosine	TH (to DOPA)	Re-uptake
		AADC (to DA)	Enzymatic (MAO, COMT)
Noradrenaline (NA)	Dopamine	DBH	Re-uptake
			Enzymatic (MAO, COMT)
Adrenaline	Noradrenaline	PNMT	Re-uptake
			Enzymatic (MAO, COMT)
Serotonin (5-HT)	Tryptophan	TPH (to 5-HTP)	Re-uptake
		AADC (to 5-HT)	Enzymatic (MAO)
Histamine	Histidine	HD	Re-uptake
			Enzymatic (MAO)
Glutamate	Glutamine	Glutaminase	Enzymatic
GABA	Glutamate	GAD	Re-uptake
			GABA shunt, GABA-T

Steps in the formation of classical neurotransmitters. AADC, amino acid decarboxylase; AChE, acetylcholinesterase; CAT, choline acetyltransferase; COMT, catechol-O-methyltransferase; DBH, dopamine β-hydroxylase; DA, dopamine; DOPA, dihydroxyphenylalanine; GABA-T, GABA transaminase; GAD, glutamic acid decarboxylase; HD, histidine decarboxylase; 5-HTP, 5-hydroxytrytophan; MAO, monoamine oxidase; PNMT, phenylethanolamine N-methyltransferase; TH, tyrosine hydroxylase; TPH, tryptophan hydroxylase.

and genetic polymorphisms (D_4 in particular). Both D_1 and D_2 receptors have wide distribution (striatal, mesolimbic and hypothalamic) while D_3 and D_4 are more localised (mesolimbic, cortical and hippocampal) (Table 1.3).

■ With regard to antipsychotic drug action:
  – The D_2 family are the important group of DA receptors.
  – The D_2 receptor is found both presynaptically (autoreceptor) and at postsynaptic sites so D_2 antagonists not only inhibit postsynaptic responses but also increase DA release by antagonism of the autoreceptor.
  – The importance of the D_4 receptor needs clarification but it shows marked polymorphism; clozapine has a high affinity for this receptor.

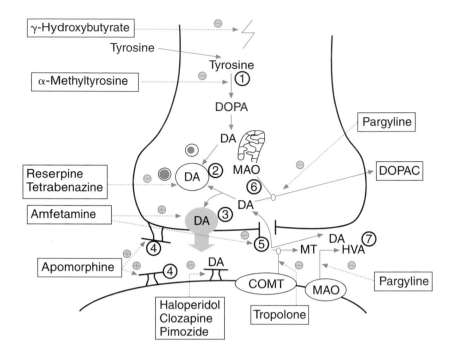

Figure 1.8 *Schematic model of a central dopaminergic neurone indicating possible sites of drug action. γ-Hydroxybutyrate effectively blocks the release of DA by blocking impulse flow in dopaminergic neurones. Tyrosine hydroxylase activity is blocked by the competitive inhibitor, α-methyltyrosine and other tyrosine hydroxylase inhibitors (1). Reserpine and tetrabenazine interfere with the uptake–storage mechanism of the amine granules. The depletion of DA produced by reserpine is long lasting and the storage granules appear to be irreversibly damaged. Tetrabenazine also interferes with the uptake storage mechanism of the granules, except that the effects of this drug do not appear to be irreversible (2). Amfetamine administered in high doses releases DA (3) but most of the releasing ability of amfetamine appears to be related to its ability to effectively block DA reuptake (5). Apomorphine is an effective DA receptor-stimulating drug, with both pre- and postsynaptic sites of action. Haloperidol, pimozide, clozapine and other antipsychotics are effective DA receptor-blocking drugs (4). DA has its action terminated by being taken up into the presynaptic terminal. Amfetamine and cocaine, as well as benztropine, an anticholinergic drug, are potent inhibitors of this re-uptake mechanism (5). DA present in a free state within the presynaptic terminal can be degraded by the enzyme monoamine oxidase (MAO) which appears to be located in the outer membrane of the mitochondria. Dihydroxyphenylacetic acid (DOPAC) is a product of the action of MAO and aldehyde oxidase on DA. Phenelzine and pargyline are inhibitors of MAO. Some MAO is also present outside the dopaminergic neurone (6). DA can be inactivated by the enzyme catechol-O-methyltransferase (COMT), which is believed to be localised outside the presynaptic neurone. Tropolone is an inhibitor of COMT (7).*

Table 1.3 *Dopamine receptors. The distribution, function, signal transduction and pharmacology of dopamine receptors in the brain*

Distribution	Functional role	D$_1$ like		*D$_2$ like		
		D$_1$	D$_5$	D$_2$	D$_3$	D$_4$
Cortex	Arousal, mood	++	–	++	–	–
Limbic system	Emotion, stereotypical behaviour	+++	–	+++	+	++
Basal ganglia	Motor control	++	+	+++	+	+
Hypothalamus	Autonomic and endocrine control	++	+	–	–	–
Pituitary gland	Endocrine control	–	–	+++	–	–
Signal transduction		Increase cAMP		Decrease cAMP and/or increase IP$_3$		
Agonists	Dopamine	+ (low potency)		+ (high potency)		
	Bromocriptine	Partial agonist				
Antagonists	Chlorpromazine	+	+	+++	+++	+
	Haloperidol	++	+	+++	+++	+++
	Clozapine	+	+	+	+	++
Effect		Mainly postsynaptic inhibition		Pre- and postsynaptic inhibition		
				Stimulation/inhibition of hormone release		

* There are short and long forms of D$_2$ receptors and variants of D$_3$ and D$_4$.

Noradrenaline (NA)

Pathways and functions

■ The principal location of NA-containing neurones is the locus coeruleus (LC) with the axons projecting up to limbic areas and descending to the spinal cord (involved in muscle co-ordination).

■ LC neurones together with those that form the ventral noradrenergic bundle project to the hypothalamus, cortex and subcortical limbic areas.
  – The cortical projections are concerned with arousal and maintaining the cortex in an alert state.
  – The limbic projections are involved in drive, motivation, mood and response to stress.

Synthesis and metabolism

■ NA is formed by the action of dopamine-β-oxidase, which converts DA to NA; drugs such as disulfram inhibit this enzyme by depleting its cofactor copper.

■ As with DA, NA is inactivated after release by re-uptake, a process inhibited by tricyclic antidepressants and venlafaxine as well as cocaine.

■ NA, like DA, is metabolised by MAO and COMT (see Table 1.2). The main CNS metabolite of NA is 3-methoxy-4-hydroxyphenylglycol (MHPG). This is in contrast to the periphery where it is vanillylmandelic acid (VMA).

■ In a manner similar to DA, NA release is under inhibitory autoreceptor (α_2) feedback regulation (Fig. 1.9)

Adrenoceptors

■ The receptors on which noradrenaline acts are divided into α- and β-adrenoceptors with further subdivisions within these two main groups.
  – Both α_1 and α_2 receptors are found within the brain at postsynaptic sites with the α_2 receptor also located on noradrenergic terminals where it acts as the autoreceptor.
  – α_1 Receptors are excitatory and use inositol phosphate as the second messenger.
  – α_2 Receptors are inhibitory and are linked to cAMP (i.e. they inhibit cAMP).
  – β-Adrenoceptors (β_1, β_2, β_3) are stimulatory and linked to cAMP (i.e. they increase cAMP).

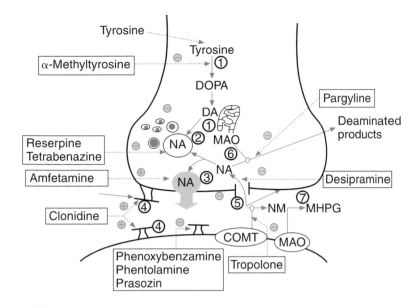

Figure 1.9 *Schematic model of central noradrenergic neurone indicating possible sites of drug action. Tyrosine hydroxylase activity is blocked by the competitive inhibitor, α-methyltyrosine while DA β-hydroxylase activity is blocked by a dithiocarbamate derivative, Fla-63 (bis-(I-methyl-4-homopiperazinyl-thiocarbonyl)-disulphide) (1). Reserpine and tetrabenazine interfere with the uptake–storage mechanism of the amine granules. The depletion of NA produced by reserpine is long lasting and the storage granules are irreversibly damaged. Tetrabenazine also interferes with the uptake–storage mechanism of the granules, except the effects of this drug are of a shorter duration and do not appear to be irreversible (2). Amfetamine appears to cause an increase in the net release of NA (3). Probably the primary mechanism by which amfetamine causes release is by its ability to effectively block the re-uptake mechanism (5). Presynaptic α$_2$-autoreceptors and postsynaptic receptors (α$_1$, α$_2$, β$_1$, β$_2$). Clonidine appears to be a very potent autoreceptor-stimulating drug. At higher doses clonidine will also stimulate postsynaptic receptors. Phenoxybenzamine and phentolamine are effective α$_1$ antagonists but may also have some presynaptic α$_2$ effects. However, yohimbine and piperoxane are more selective as α$_2$ antagonists (4). NA has its action terminated by uptake. The tricyclic drug desipramine is an example of a potent inhibitor of this uptake mechanism as well as the newer SNRIs (venlafaxine) and cocaine (5). NA or DA present in a free state within the presynaptic terminal can be degraded by the enzyme MAO, which appears to be located in the outer membrane of mitochondria. Pargyline is an effective inhibitor of MAO (6). NA can be inactivated by the membrane-bound enzyme catechol-O-methyltransferase (COMT). Tropolone is an inhibitor of COMT. The normetanephrine (NM) formed by the action of COMT on NE can be further metabolised by MAO to 3-methoxy-4-hydroxyphenylglycol (MHPG) (7).*

Serotonin (5-hydroxytryptamine; 5-HT)

Pathways and functions

■ The neurones containing 5-HT are located in the midbrain and brainstem raphe nuclei from where extend long ascending (dorsal and median raphe) or descending (obscurus, magnus and pallidus raphe nuclei) pathways.

■ The ascending pathways innervate the hippocampus (mainly from the median raphe), striatum, amygdala and hypothalamus (mainly dorsal raphe).

– They have a wide modulatory role in various aspects of behaviour including mood and emotion, sleep/wakefulness and regulation of circadian functions (suprachiasmatic nucleus), control of consummatory behaviours (feeding, sex), body temperature, perceptions (hallucinations – LSD is a 5-HT_{2A} receptor agonist) and vomiting (5-HT_3 receptor antagonists (e.g. ondansetron, are anti-emetic).

■ The descending pathways:

– terminate in the dorsal horn of the spinal cord where they are involved in the inhibition of pain transmission; and

– the ventral horn where they regulate motor neurone output.

Synthesis and metabolism

■ 5-HT is formed by the hydroxylation of tryptophan, by tryptophan hydroxylase, to 5-hydroxytryptophan (5 HTP), followed by decarboxylation to 5-HT using 5-HTP decarboxylase, which is the same enzyme as DOPA decarboxylase (see Table 1.2).

■ Importantly, brain tryptophan hydroxylase is unsaturated at normal concentrations of tryptophan in the brain, hence altering availability of brain tryptophan will alter brain 5-HT levels.

■ Tryptophan enters the brain by the large neutral amino acid-facilitated transport system, which is competitive. Thus it is possible to lower brain 5-HT either by reducing plasma tryptophan or by 'flooding' the transport carrier with another large neutral amino acid such as valine. This is the basis of the studies using the manipulation of tryptophan levels in humans to investigate the function of brain 5-HT.

■ Various amfetamines, such as parachloroamfetamine, fenfluramine and MDMA (Ecstasy), cause the release of terminal 5-HT.

■ The major mechanism for removing 5-HT from the synaptic cleft is re-uptake by the 5-HT transporter, which is inhibited by re-uptake inhibitors (SSRIs and tricyclic antidepressants).

- 5-HT is also metabolised by MAO to form 5-hydroxyindole acetic acid (5-HIAA), which is actively transported across the blood-brain barrier out of the brain, in common with other low molecular weight organic acids (e.g. HVA, uric acid).
- 5-HT release at the terminals is subject to inhibitory autoregulation involving the 5-HT$_{1B/D}$ receptor (Fig. 1.10).

5-HT receptors

- There are 14 5-HT receptors, all are G-protein coupled apart from 5-HT$_3$ (ligand-gated cation channel).
- The 5-HT$_1$ group, (5-HT$_{1A}$, 5-HT$_{1B}$, 5-HT$_{1D}$) are inhibitory and are negatively coupled to cAMP.

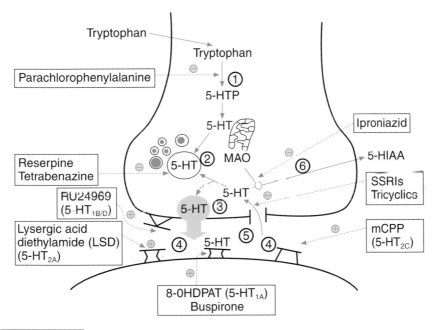

Figure 1.10 Schematic model of a central serotonergic neurone indicating possible sites of drug action. Tryptophan is converted to 5-hydroxytryptophan (5-HTP) by tryptophan hydroxylase (1) and this enzyme can be inhibited by parachlorophenylalanine (pCPA) but this compound has only experimental value. 5-HTP is then converted to 5-HT and stored in vesicles (2), a process disrupted by reserpine and tetrabenazine. 5-HT is released by a Ca^{2+}-dependent process (3); parachloramfetamine and fenfluramine increase 5-HT release while activation of 5-HT$_{1B/D}$ autoreceptors inhibits release (at the cell bodies this function is served by 5-HT$_{1A}$ receptors). After release 5-HT activates a range of postsynaptic 5-HT receptors (4) to produce functional responses and behavioural outcomes. After release 5-HT is either taken up again into the terminal, stored and re-used (5) or metabolised to 5-hydroxyindole acetic acid (5-HIAA) by MAO (6). The SSRIs and tricyclics prevent re-uptake.

- The 5-HT_{1A} receptor is found both at presynaptic (somatodendritic autoreceptor) and postsynaptic sites including the hippocampus and periaqueductal grey (PAG) where importantly it regulates behaviours such as resilience, impulsivity and restraint of excessive response to stress. The 5-HT_{1A} receptor may be an important target in the action of antidepressants.

■ 5-HT_2 receptors (5-HT_{2A}, 5-HT_{2B}, 5-HT_{2C}) are excitatory and act through the phospholipase C/inositol phosphate pathway.

- 5-HT_{2A} receptors are found in the cortex and are associated with sensory perception.
- 5-HT_{2C} receptors when activated reduce food intake and induce anxiety/panic.

■ The 5-HT_4, 5-HT_5, 5-HT_6 and 5-HT_7 receptors are positively coupled to cAMP and are thus excitatory. 5-HT_6 receptor antagonists have been shown, in animal studies, to increase aspects of memory, in particular retention of information and attention, while the 5-HT_7 receptor may have importance in depression and circadian functions (suprachiasmatic nucleus) (Fig.1.11).

Acetylcholine (ACh)

Pathways and functions

■ The distribution of ACh in the brain is more diffuse than that of the catecholamines and 5-HT.

■ The neurones are located in the mid- and hindbrain. The most important pathway with regard to psychopharmacology has cell bodies in the nucleus basalis of Meynert with axons innervating the hippocampus. This pathway is disrupted in Alzheimer's disease and is probably associated with the consequent memory dysfunction.

Synthesis and metabolism

■ ACh is formed by the enzymatic (choline acetyltransferase) conversion of choline and acetyl coenzyme-A (CoA) to ACh (see Table 1.2 and Fig. 1.12).

■ Following release ACh is metabolised by acetylcholine esterase (AChE) to form choline. Choline is taken up into the neurone by an active transport system and can then be re-used to sythesise ACh.

■ Drugs that inhibit AChE are used in the symptomatic treatment of Alzheimer's disease (see Chapter 9).

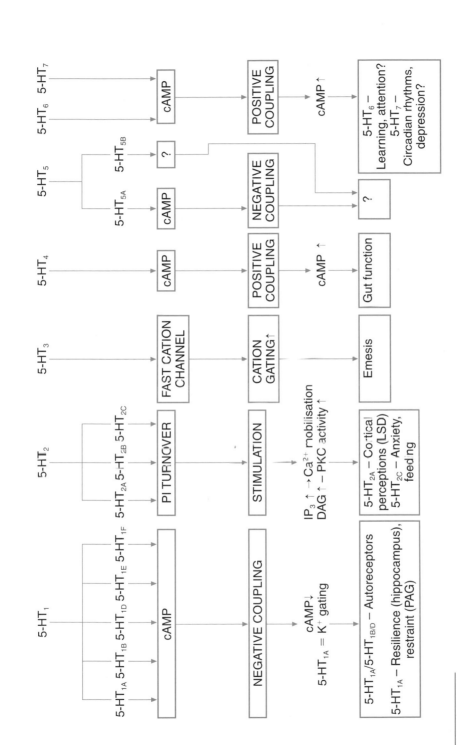

Figure 1.11 Summary diagram of the types of 5-HT receptors, their receptor coupling mechanisms and proposed functions.

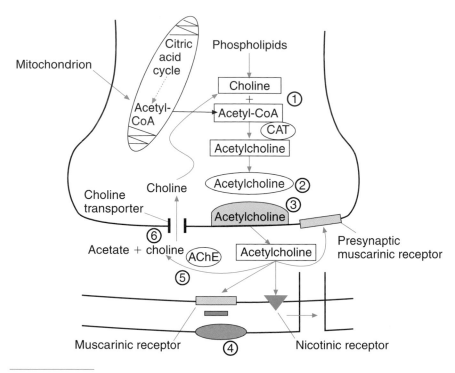

Figure 1.12 *Schematic model of a central cholinergic nerve ending indicating possible sites of drug action. Attempts have been made to increase acetycholine synthesis (CAT = choline acetyltransferase) by increasing availability of choline but this has not been successful (1). ACh is stored in vesicles but there are no clinically effective drugs that act at this site (2). There is some evidence that aminopyridines and phosphatidylserines release ACh and may have limited use in Alzheimer's disease patients (3). Muscarinic antagonists are used for Parkinson's disease and antipsychotic-induced extrapyramidal side-effects. Presynaptic muscarinic autoreceptors reduce ACh release and may be a future target for drug action. Existing agonists (e.g. for Alzheimer's disease) have poor brain penetration and short half-lives (4). Acetylcholinesterase is a major drug target for the symptomatic treatment of Alzheimer's disease. Some recent esterase inhibitors show limited promise with lower incidence of autonomic side-effects (5). Choline is transported back into the neurone and re-used (6).*

Cholinergic receptors

■ These are subdivided into two classes: nicotinic and muscarinic, with further subdivision within the classes.

■ Nicotinic receptors are involved in fast excitatory synaptic transmission and are directly coupled to cation channels. These receptors are divided into two basic types: muscle ganglionic and central nervous system (CNS), with the CNS type widespread in the brain and variable with respect to their molecular composition and location.

■ There are five muscarinic receptors (M_1–M_5) which are G-protein coupled and either activate formation of IP_3 (M_1, M_3, M_5) or inhibit cAMP (M_2, M_4).

They are all found in the brain, and agonists at certain of these receptors (e.g. M_1) offer potential targets for the treatment of Alzheimer's disease but without much success as yet (poor brain penetration, short half-lives and effects outside the CNS).

γ-Aminobutyric acid (GABA)

■ GABA neurones are widely distributed within the brain with the highest densities in the basal ganglia, hypothalamus, amygdala and other limbic areas.

■ GABA is formed by decarboxylation of glutamate using the enzyme glutamate decarboxylase.

■ Following release GABA can either be taken up into the nerve terminals by a specific transport system or it enters glial cells where it undergoes mitochondrial metabolism back to glutamate (*GABA shunt*) (see Table 1.2).

■ The major psychopharmacological interest in GABA is the role of the $GABA_A$ receptor complex in the action of benzodiazepines, barbiturates, alcohol and neurosteroids (Fig. 1.13 and see Chapter 6).

■ The receptor is directly coupled to a chloride ion channel and activation results in an influx of chloride ions and rapid hyperpolarisation (causing inhibition).

■ Barbiturates lock the channel open resulting in prolonged irreversible neuronal inhibition. They can act in the absence of GABA and hence their toxicity in overdose (respiratory depression).

■ The benzodiazepines bind to a site on the $GABA_A$ receptor complex and facilitate the action of GABA so increasing the frequency of chloride channel opening. Because they require GABA to be present for their action they are less toxic in overdose than barbiturates.

  – Benzodiazepines are agonists at their binding sites and their actions can be blocked by antagonists (e.g. flumazenil) while inverse-agonists at the benzodiazepine site decrease GABA transmission (see Fig 1.13).

  – Newer hypnotics such as zopiclone have similar actions to benzodiazepines but interact with specific subunits of the $GABA_A$ receptor which may reduce the adverse effects (memory loss, dependence).

■ There are also $GABA_B$ receptors in the brain found at both pre- and postsynaptic sites. These receptors increase K^+ conductance and produce slow inhibitory potentials through inhibition of cAMP. The physiological and behavioural significance of these receptors is not well understood but they

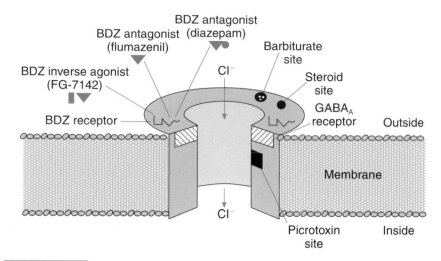

Figure 1.13 *GABA is the major inhibitory neurotransmitter, with two types of receptor. This figure shows the GABA$_A$ receptor. Activation of the GABA$_A$ receptor leads to an influx of Cl$^-$ ions (hyperpolarisation). It is composed of subunits which have heterogeneous distribution in the brain and which may offer selective drug targets (i.e. removal of the α_1 subunit has no effect on anxiolytic effects of benzodiazepines but results in loss of the sedative and anti-epileptic effects). The GABA$_A$ receptor is part of a complex with multiple binding sites (benzodiazepine (BDZ), steroid, barbiturate, etc.). Benzodiazepines are agonists at a site which modulates the ability of GABA to bind to its site. Agonists at this site facilitate GABA binding whereas inverse agonists reduce it, resulting in stimulatory effects. Barbiturates bind directly to the Cl$^-$ ion channel. Bicuculline is an antagonist of the GABA$_A$ binding site while muscimol is an agonist at that site. Picrotoxin acts as a channel blocker.*

may be important in absence seizures, cognitive performance and the regulation of amine release.

Glutamate

■ This is the major fast-acting excitatory neurotransmitter with a wide distribution in the brain. There are four main types of excitatory amino acid receptors: N-methyl D-aspartate (NMDA), amino-3-hydroxy-5-methyl-4-isoxazole propionate (AMPA), kainate (these all regulate cation channels) and metabotropic (G-protein coupled). There are many subtypes within these groups.

■ There are two major reasons for the growing interest in brain glutamate:
  – firstly, the link between glutamate (NMDA) receptor activation and long-term potentiation (LTP) in the hippocampus as the physiological substrate of memory;

– secondly, the link between excessive glutamate receptor activation and neurodegeneration caused by loss of intracellular Ca^{2+} homeostasis.

■ There is also interest in the role of glutamate transmission in psychosis (schizophrenia) and anxiety. Antagonists at glutamate receptors have yet to be developed for clinical use. Ketamine and phencyclidine (PCP) and dizocilpine (MK801) block the channel of the NMDA receptor.

■ Ionotropic glutamate receptors:
  – These include the NMDA receptor, which has attracted most attention.
  – The NMDA receptor (Fig. 1.14) is a complex structure with several regulatory sites apart from the glutamate-binding site.
  – Activation of the receptor can lead to changes in Na^+, Ca^{2+} and K^+ conductance through the channel; drugs such as dizocilpine and PCP bind in the channel acting as antagonists.
  – Both LTP and excitotoxicity are associated with NMDA receptor activation.

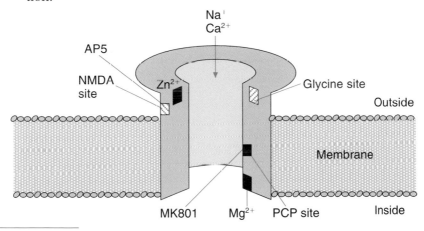

Figure 1.14 *Diagram of the N-methyl D-aspartate (NMDA) ionotropic glutamate receptor linked to a Na^+ channel. The diagram shows the glutamate/NMDA binding site and some of the numerous other regulatory sites on this receptor. Glycine is a co-agonist at this receptor. Activation of this receptor is accompanied by an influx of Ca^{2+}. Drugs such as ketamine, MK801 and phencyclidine (PCP) act as antagonists at the NMDA receptor by blocking the channel. At resting, membrane potential magnesium (Mg^{2+}) voltage dependently blocks the channel; this is removed when the membrane is depolarised. 2-amino-5-phosphopentanoic acid (AP5) is an NMDA antagonist. Zinc (Zn^{2+}) binds to a divalent cation site to produce a voltage-independent block of the channel.*

■ Metabotropic glutamate receptors:
  – Activation causes formation of IP_3 and release of Ca^{2+} which may have a role in glutamate excitotoxicity and synaptic plasticity.
  – Development of metabotropic receptor antagonists may offer an approach to the development of neuroprotective drugs.

References

Further reading

Bear MF, Connors BW, Paradiso MA. Neuroscience Exploring the Brain, 2nd edn. Baltimore: Lippincott, Williams & Wilkins, 2001. (Little on drugs.)

Cooper JR, Bloom FE, Roth RH. The Biochemical Basis of Neuropharmacology, 8th edn. Oxford (NY): Oxford University Press, 2003.

Hammond C. Cellular and Molecular Neurobiology, 2nd edn. London: Academic Press, 2001. (Neurotransmitter receptor mechanisms.)

Leonard BE. Fundamentals of Psychopharmacology, 3rd edn. Chichester: John Wiley, 2003.

Rang HP, Dale MM, Ritter JM, Moore PK. Pharmacology, 5th edn. Edinburgh: Churchill Livingstone, 2003. (Pharmacology, not specifically psychopharmacology.)

2 Pharmacokinetics and pharmacodynamics

Pharmacokinetics

Basics

- Pharmacokinetics is concerned with the time-course and disposition of drugs in the body ('the body's effect on drugs').
- Drugs are intended to act on target organs but usually have to be given systemically.
- *Bioavailability* (how much of an administered drug reaches its target) is determined by three main factors:
  - absorption;
  - distribution;
  - elimination (metabolism and/or excretion).
- The *law of mass action* states that 'the rate of a reaction is proportional to the active masses of the reacting substances'. This results in:
- *First-order kinetics* (Fig. 2.1) where the rate of absorption or elimination is directly proportional to the amount of drug remaining (for nonreversible reactions). This applies to most psychopharmacological drugs.
- With *zero-order kinetics* (see Fig. 2.1) a fixed amount of drug is absorbed or eliminated for each unit of time independent of drug concentrations, because of some other rate-limiting factor. Examples are the metabolism of alcohol and phenytoin (saturation of metabolic enzymes) and absorption of controlled-release drugs and depot antipsychotics.

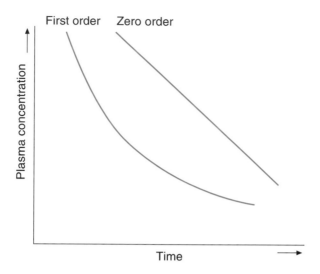

Figure 2.1 *In elimination with zero-order kinetics, concentration falls steadily in a straight line, whereas with first-order kinetics the curve is exponential.*

Figure 2.2 shows the hypothetical plasma concentration after drug administration.

- Following drug administration, there is a rise and fall in plasma concentration determined by the processes of absorption, distribution and elimination.
- C_{max} is the maximum plasma concentration achieved.
- t_{max} is the time to maximum (peak) plasma concentration.
- $t_{1/2}$ is the time for the plasma concentration to fall by a half (elimination half-life), in this case by first-order kinetics.
- The area under the curve (AUC) after a single dose is proportional to the amount of drug in plasma and allows determination of fraction of dose absorbed – the bioavailability.

Different routes of administration and relevant features are described in Table 2.1.

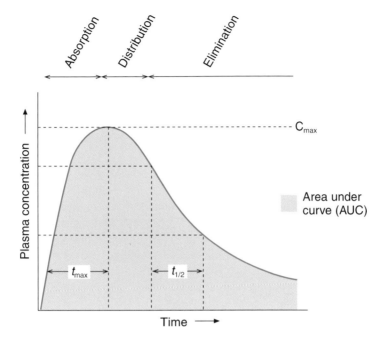

Figure 2.2 *Plasma drug concentration in the phases of absorption, distribution and elimination.*

Absorption

■ Absorption is influenced by the route of administration and drug properties.

■ Drug delivery systems allow modification of absorption (e.g. enteric coating or delayed-release tablets, depot preparations).

■ Liquid preparations (e.g. risperidone, fluoxetine) and oral dispersible tablets (e.g. olanzapine, risperidone, mirtazapine) are aimed at ensuring administration/improving compliance. They generally have minimal effects on absorption.

Table 2.1 *Comparison of routes of drug administration*

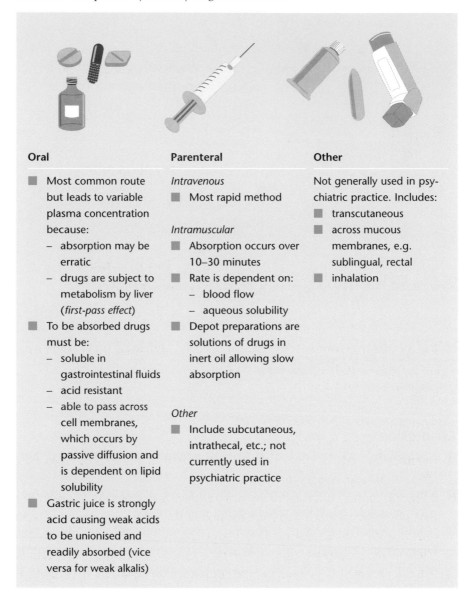

Oral

- Most common route but leads to variable plasma concentration because:
  - absorption may be erratic
  - drugs are subject to metabolism by liver (*first-pass effect*)
- To be absorbed drugs must be:
  - soluble in gastrointestinal fluids
  - acid resistant
  - able to pass across cell membranes, which occurs by passive diffusion and is dependent on lipid solubility
- Gastric juice is strongly acid causing weak acids to be unionised and readily absorbed (vice versa for weak alkalis)

Parenteral

Intravenous
- Most rapid method

Intramuscular
- Absorption occurs over 10–30 minutes
- Rate is dependent on:
  - blood flow
  - aqueous solubility
- Depot preparations are solutions of drugs in inert oil allowing slow absorption

Other
- Include subcutaneous, intrathecal, etc.; not currently used in psychiatric practice

Other

Not generally used in psychiatric practice. Includes:
- transcutaneous
- across mucous membranes, e.g. sublingual, rectal
- inhalation

Distribution (Fig. 2.3)

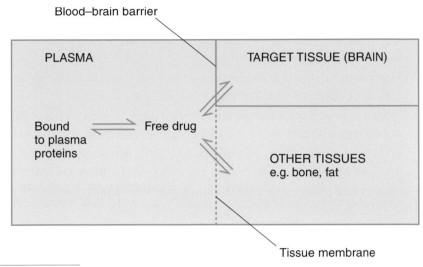

Figure 2.3 *Distribution of drug between different body 'compartments'.*

■ During the (re)distribution phase in plasma the drug is distributed to various tissues in the body depending on:
 – plasma protein binding;
 – tissue perfusion;
 – permeability of tissue membranes;
 – active transport out of tissues (P-glycoprotein).
■ Distribution leads to a fall in plasma concentration and is most rapid after intravenous administration.
■ Distribution can be viewed as the drug achieving equilibrium between different 'compartments'. An approximation is the two-compartment model: central compartment (plasma) and peripheral compartment (tissues).
■ The apparent volume of distribution ($V_d = Q/C_p$) tells us about the characteristics of a drug (V_d = volume of distribution; Q = quantity of drug; C_p = plasma concentration). When V_d is high it indicates that the drug has a high affinity for tissues outside body water such as brain and fat.
■ Drugs may be bound to sites where they exert no effect but which influence distribution and elimination:
 – Plasma proteins – if highly bound to these, drugs (e.g. many antidepressants, anticonvulsants and warfarin) may displace each other leading to increased free plasma concentration.

- Fat and other sites which may only release drugs slowly leading to persistence of drugs in the body (e.g. antipsychotics).
■ The blood-brain barrier is a consequence of the special nature of capillaries in the brain and only allows lipid-soluble molecules into the brain (most psychotropic drugs are lipid soluble):
  - Non-lipid-soluble drugs require special transport systems which can be active (e.g. L-tryptophan, L-dopa) or passive (e.g. lithium).
  - P-glycoprotein is an endothelial membrane protein which pumps drugs out of capillary cells by an ATP-dependent process and effectively prevents some drugs getting into the brain (e.g. the opioid loperamide).
  - Areas of brain not protected by the blood-brain barrier include the median eminence of the hypothalamus and the vomiting centre.

Elimination (Fig. 2.4)

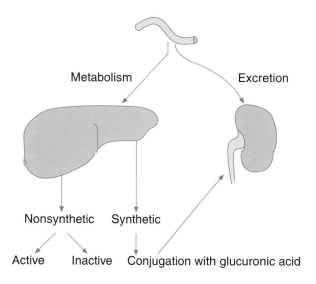

Figure 2.4 *Routes of elimination of a drug.*

Metabolism
■ Metabolism by the liver is most important but it may also occur in plasma, lung and kidney.
■ Metabolism may be to active compounds (sometimes called phase I) or to inactive compounds (phase II).
■ Nonsynthetic reactions:
  - Consist of oxidation, reduction, hydrolysis.

- May produce inactive or active compounds.
- The cytochrome P450 (CYP450) family of hepatic enzymes are responsible for oxidative metabolism of most psychotropic drugs.
- The most important isoenzymes and examples of their metabolites are:

    2D6 – typical antipsychotics, tricyclic antidepressants, paroxetine, fluoxetine;

    3A4 – tricyclic antidepressants, carbamazepine, benzodiazepines, CA^{2+}-channel blockers;

    1A2 – tricyclic antidepressants, haloperidol, clozapine;

    2C9 – phenytoin, warfarin, fluoxetine;

    2C19 – diazepam, tricyclic antidepressants.
- There is genetic variation in hepatic enzymes affecting rate of metabolism. The most studied is CYP450-2D6; 5–10% of Caucasians, but only 1–2% of Asians, lack this enzyme and are poor metabolisers of the probe drug substrate, dextromethorphan. There are also extensive metabolisers of dextromethorphan.

Synthetic reactions (conjugation):
- Usually with glucuronic acid.
- Produce inactive, water-soluble compounds.

Factors influencing metabolism:
- Genetic variation in the activity of CYP450 enzymes (see above).
- Drug interactions leading to the inhibition or induction of CYP450 enzymes (resulting in decreased and increased metabolism respectively). Examples of isoenzyme inhibition by psychotropic drugs:

    2D6 – paroxetine, fluoxetine, tricyclic antidepressants, antipsychotics;

    3A4 – fluoxetine, nefazodone;

    1A2 – fluvoxamine;

    2C19 – fluvoxamine, fluoxetine.

    Examples of CYP450 isoenzyme induction by psychotropic drugs:

    3A3/4 – carbamazepine, phenytoin;

    2C9 – phenobarbitone;

    2C19 – carbamazepine.
- Drugs competing for same metabolic pathway (decreasing metabolism of both).
- Impaired liver function due to increased age, liver impairment (decreases metabolism).

Excretion

■ Excretion by the kidneys is most important but it may occur through the lungs or in bile, sweat, milk and saliva.
■ May be of active drug or its metabolites:
  – Ionised and non-lipid-soluble compounds are excreted best.
  – Lithium is the most important drug primarily excreted by the kidneys.
■ Factors influencing excretion:
  – Reduction in renal blood flow (nonsteroidal anti-inflammatory drugs, dehydration).
  – Alteration in reabsorption (urine pH, e.g. alkaline diuresis reduces aspirin reabsorption and increases excretion; low Na^+ increases lithium reabsorption and decreases excretion).
  – Decreased renal function due to renal impairment, increased age (decreases excretion).

Elimination half-life and steady-state concentration (Fig. 2.5)

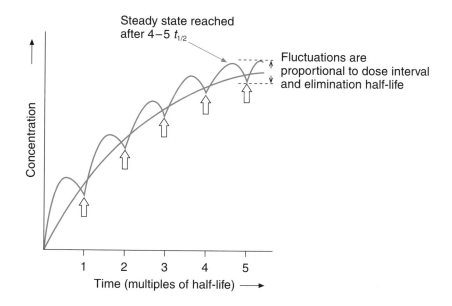

Figure 2.5 *Plasma concentration of a drug after repeated administration.*

■ *Steady-state concentration* is achieved after repeated doses lead to an equilibrium between absorption and elimination:
  – This is dependent on dose, time between doses and elimination half-life.
  – It is achieved after 4–5 half-lives; doses given at greater intervals than the half-life lead to large fluctuations in plasma concentration.
  – Delayed release preparations which slow absorption are an attempt to reduce plasma fluctuations with daily dosing (e.g. venlafaxine, lithium) or to allow long intervals between administrations (e.g. depot antipsychotics).
■ Large initial doses (*loading doses*) may be given to achieve therapeutic plasma concentrations more rapidly (e.g. sodium valproate in mania).
■ Some drugs have a recognised *therapeutic range* of plasma concentrations (e.g. lithium).
■ The *therapeutic index* is the ratio of the minimum plasma drug concentration causing toxic effects to that causing a therapeutic effect. A low therapeutic index (e.g. lithium, phenytoin) usually requires monitoring of plasma/serum concentrations.

Pharmacodynamics

Basics
■ Pharmacodynamics is the study of the mechanism of drug action ('the effect of drugs on the body').
■ Most psychoactive drugs affect the function of specific neurotransmitters either directly or indirectly (see below).
■ Drugs affecting monoamine neurotransmitters, DA, NA, 5-HT, are important in the treatment of psychotic and affective disorders.
■ Drugs acting on amino acid neurotransmitters, GABA and glutamate are important in the treatment of anxiety disorders and epilepsy.
■ There is increasing interest in drugs acting on other neurotransmitters (e.g. peptides, nitric oxide).
■ Alteration of neurotransmitter function is also commonly responsible for side-effects (unwanted or adverse effects).
■ Drugs may also act at sites that directly alter neuronal function (e.g. anaesthetics, alcohol).

Sites of drug action on neurotransmitters (Fig. 2.6)

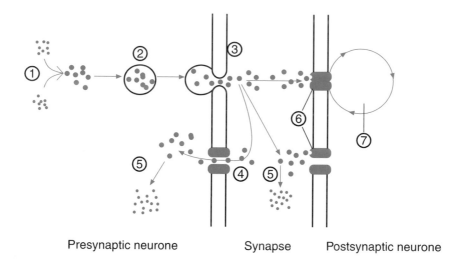

Presynaptic neurone · Synapse · Postsynaptic neurone

Figure 2.6 *Sites of drug action on neurotransmitters (for key to numbers see text).*

1. *Synthesis* (e.g. L-tryptophan is the precursor of 5-HT and administration results in increased 5-HT synthesis).
2. *Storage* (e.g. reserpine depletes NA and DA stores in nerve terminal vesicles).
3. *Release* (e.g. amphetamine releases NA and DA into the synapse).
4. *Re-uptake* (e.g. TCAs inhibit monoamine re-uptake into the presynaptic neurone and so increase neurotransmitter concentration in the synapse).
5. *Degradation* (e.g. monoamine oxidase inhibitors, MAOIs, prevent the breakdown of monoamine neurotransmitters).
6. *Receptors* (e.g. antipsychotics antagonise DA receptors).
7. *Other postsynaptic mechanisms* (e.g. lithium inhibits second messenger function, Ca^{2+} channel antagonists).

Agonists

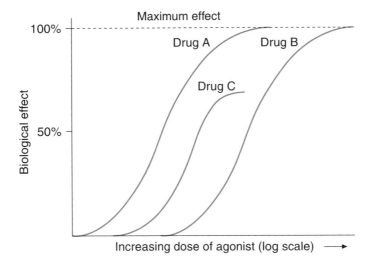

Figure 2.7 Different pattern of responses to agonists.

■ *Agonists* are drugs that mimic endogenous neurotransmitters.
■ Most drugs bind reversibly to receptors and in the simplest case the response is proportional to the fraction of receptors occupied (*law of mass action*).
■ As the concentration of a drug increases the response increases until all the receptors are occupied giving a *dose–response curve* as shown in Fig. 2.7. When maximum effects are achieved without full receptor occupancy there are said to be *spare receptors*.
■ In Fig. 2.7 the two *full agonists* (A and B) are able to bring about maximum responses, however A does so at a lower concentration than B because it has a greater *affinity* for the receptor.
■ Drug C in Fig. 2.7 has a lower *efficacy* than A and B and does not cause a maximal response even when all receptors are occupied, and is a partial agonist (e.g. buspirone, buprenorphine, aripiprazole). Partial agonists can partially antagonise the effect of full agonist (see below).
■ The *potency* of a drug is determined by:
    – the proportion of the drug reaching the receptor;
    – its affinity for the receptor;
    – its efficacy.

Antagonists

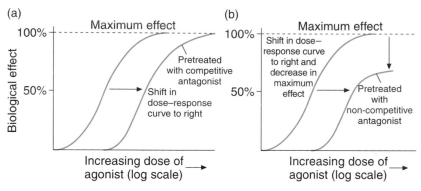

Figure 2.8 *Effect of antagonists on the action of agonist drugs.*

■ *Antagonists* bind to receptors without causing an effect and they block the action of agonists causing a reduced effect for a given concentration of agonist (shift to the right in the dose–response curve for the agonist).

■ Most antagonist drugs are *competitive* and are displaced from their binding sites by agonists so that at high doses the agonist can still exert maximum effect (Fig. 2.8a). This competition is influenced by the relative affinity of the agonist and antagonist for the receptor.

■ *Noncompetitive antagonists* cannot be displaced by agonists and not only shift the curve to the right but also reduce the maximum effect (Fig. 2.8b). Noncompetitive antagonists may be reversible if the system is restored to normal when the antagonist is removed, or irreversible if restoration of function requires synthesis of new receptors.

■ In the presence of a full agonist, increasing concentrations of a partial agonist will antagonise the response until the level of its intrinsic activity is reached (Fig. 2.9). Higher doses of a high-affinity partial agonist there-fore 'set' a level of neurotransmission which is independent of the concen-tration of agonist (e.g. it is proposed that aripiprazole '*stabilises*' DA neurotransmission, avoiding both over- and underactivity, resulting in benefit to both positive and negative symptoms of schizophrenia without causing extrapyramidal side-effects).

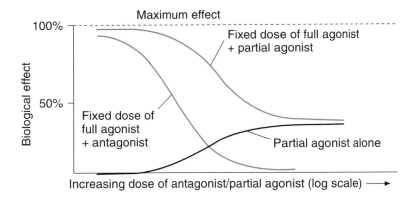

Figure 2.9 *Effect of increasing doses of a partial agonist, alone, and in the presence of a full agonist.*

Tolerance and sensitisation

■ *Tolerance* describes the diminished response to the administration of a drug after repeated exposure. It may be caused by:

– increased metabolism (e.g. carbamazepine increases the activity of enzymes that metabolise it: *enzyme induction*);

– reduced receptor sensitivity or number (*downregulation*);

– activation of a homeostatic mechanism (e.g. in the second messenger or effector system);

– behavioural tolerance through learning to cope with the effects.

■ *Cross-tolerance* between drugs is the basis for a number of drug interactions (e.g. alcohol with barbiturates; carbamazepine with oral contraceptives).

■ *Sensitisation* is the enhancement of drug effects following the repeated administration of the same dose of drug (e.g. stimulants such as amphetamines in animals).

References

Further reading
Cooper JR, Bloom FE, Roth RH. The Biochemical Basis of Neuropharmacology, 8th edn. Oxford (NY): Oxford University Press, 2003
Feldman RS, Meyer JS, Quenzer LF. Principles of Neuropsychopharmacology. Sunderland (MA): Sinauer Associates, 1997
King J (ed). Seminars in Clinical Psychopharmacology. London: Gaskell, 1995 (new edition imminent)
Schatzberg AF, Nemeroff CB. The American Psychiatric Publishing Textbook of Psychopharmacology, 3rd edn. Arlington: APPI, 2004
Shiloh R, Nutt D, Weizman A. Atlas of Psychiatric Pharmacotherapy. London: Martin Dunitz, 1999

3 Antipsychotics

History

Like the antidepressants, antipsychotic drugs were discovered by chance.

- *1950s*: Phenothiazines developed. Chlorpromazine was synthesised originally as an antihistamine/antihelminthic but was found subsequently to be sedative and antipsychotic. More compounds were synthesised within the same and related classes (e.g. thioxanthines; Table 3.1). The butyrophenones were created in the late 1950s: haloperidol began life as a candidate analgesic, and was later found to have antipsychotic properties. Further compounds were synthesised in this and other classes, e.g. phenyl butylpiperidine.
- *1970s*: Atypicals developed (Table 3.2). Classified 'atypical' on the basis of reduced extrapyramidal side-effects in animal models (e.g. thioridazine, sulpiride).
- *1980s*: Clozapine 'rediscovered' with recognition of broader efficacy compared with other antipsychotics.
- *1990s*: New-generation atypical antipsychotics introduced: amisulpride, olanzapine, quetiapine, risperidone, sertindole, ziprasidone.
- *2000s*: First partial DA agonist antipsychotic introduced: aripiprazole.

The dopamine hypothesis

The DA system (see Chapter 1) is believed to play an important role in the action of antipsychotic drugs.

- Antipsychotics increase turnover of brain DA.

■ The greater the DA receptor binding affinity of an antipsychotic, the greater the clinical potency (Fig. 3.1).

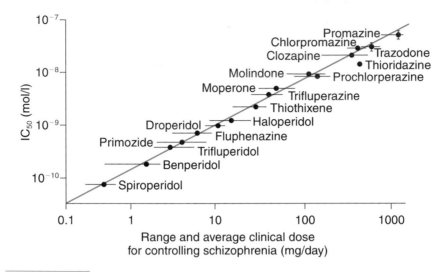

Figure 3.1 Affinity for DA receptors and clinical potency. Source: Reprinted with permission from Creese *et al.* 1976. Copyright © 1976, American Association for the Advancement of Science.

■ α- but not β-flupenthixol has antipsychotic activity greater than placebo (only the α isomer is antagonist at D_2 receptors) (Fig. 3.2).

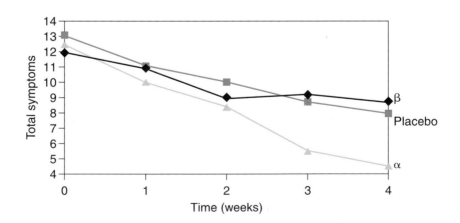

Figure 3.2 Efficacy of α- and β-flupenthixol in schizophrenia. The α-isomer caused a greater improvement in symptomatology than placebo while the β-isomer was without antipsychotic efficacy. Source: Reproduced with permission from Johnstone *et al.* 1978.

■ Enhanced amphetamine-induced release of DA in patients with schizophrenia compared with controls using single photon emission computerised tomography (SPECT) imaging, implies presynaptic DA system
abnormalities in schizophrenia (Fig. 3.3).

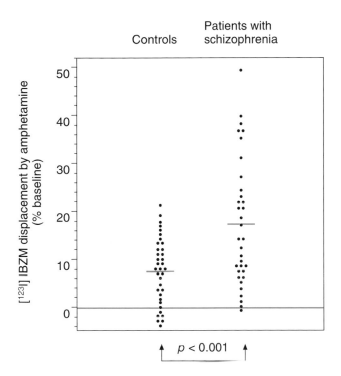

Figure 3.3 *Dopamine transmission and schizophrenia. This graph illustrates the effect
of amphetamine (0.3 mg/kg) on [^{123}I]IBZM binding in healthy control subjects and
untreated patients with schizophrenia. The results indicate that when challenged with
amphetamine, patients with schizophrenia release more dopamine than healthy controls.
The amount of release is related to the increase in positive symptoms.* Source: Reproduced
with permission from Laruelle *et al.* 1996.

■ *Late 1990s*: Series of neurochemical imaging experiments indicates that
above approx. 60% of striatal D$_2$-like receptor occupancy predicts antipsychotic efficacy whilst greater than approx. 80% predicts the onset of
extrapyramidal side-effects (EPSE) (Fig. 3.4).

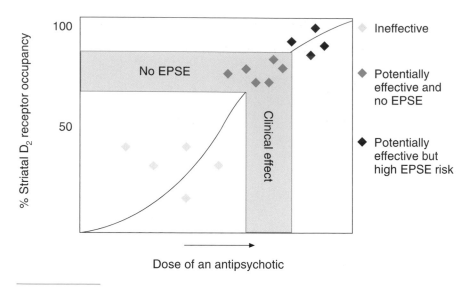

Figure 3.4 *D$_2$-like receptor occupancy levels, clinical efficacy and side-effects. D$_2$ receptor occupancy between 60–80% is associated with efficacy with minimal extrapyramidal side-effects (EPSE).*

Role of dopamine receptor subtypes

(see also Chapter 1)

Although typical and most atypical antipsychotics have many different pharmacological effects, they share the property of blocking the D$_2$ receptor subtype. However:

- 20–50% of patients do not respond to D$_2$ antagonists.
- Some atypical antipsychotics achieve an antipsychotic effect without high D$_2$ occupancy.
- No consistent evidence from positron emission tomography (PET) studies or genetic association studies to suggest a constitutional change in D$_2$ receptors in schizophrenia.

The role of D$_3$ and D$_4$ receptor subtypes is also uncertain:

- Some atypical antipsychotics have a high affinity for D$_3$ and D$_4$ receptors.
- D$_3$ and D$_4$ receptors are distributed in proportionately higher densities in limbic areas.
- Genetic association studies suggest that abnormal D$_3$ variants (but not D$_4$ variants) may occur in excess in patients with schizophrenia.
- Some post-mortem studies suggest that D$_3$ and D$_4$ receptor densities may be greater in the schizophrenic brain.

■ However, some D_4 antagonists do not have antipsychotic properties.

Table 3.1 *Chemical classification of typical antipsychotics*

Phenothiazines	Aliphatic side-chains	Chlorpromazine
	Piperidine	Thioridazine (restricted use due to ↑QTc)
	Piperazine	Trifluperazine
		Fluphenazine
Thioxanthenes		Flupentixol
		Zuclopenthixol
Butyrophenones		Haloperidol
		Droperidol (withdrawn due to ↑QTc)
Diphenylbutylpiperidines		Pimozide
Substituted benzamides		Sulpiride (NB sulpiride is considered by some to be an atypical antipsychotic)

Table 3.2 *Chemical classification of atypical antipsychotics*

Dibenzodiazepines	Clozapine
Thienobenzodiazepine	Olanzapine
Dibenzothiazepine	Quetiapine
Benzixasoles	Risperidone
Imidazolidinone	Sertindole (monitoring required for ↑QTc)
Substituted benzamides	Amisulpride
Quinolinones	Aripiprazole

Table 3.3 *Clinical indications for antipsychotics*

Psychiatric	Non-psychiatric
Treatment of psychosis	Nausea
Treatment of mania	Anaesthesia (neuroleptanalgesia, premedication)
Sedation/tranquillisation	Intractable hiccough
Severe anxiety	Terminal illness
? Depression	

Therapeutic actions of antipsychotic drugs

The chemical classification of older or newer antipsychotics is given in Tables 3.1 and 3.2 and their clinical uses in Table 3.3. Given that each of the newer antipsychotics belongs to a different chemical class, attention has turned to delineating their different pharmaceutical properties. In the UK the National Institute for Clinical Excellence (NICE) has given guidance on the use of atypical antipsychotics in schizophrenia (Technology Appraisal No. 43, 2002) recommending their use as first-line treatment. NICE has issued general guidelines for the treatment of schizophrenia (NICE, 2002) including acute behavioural disturbance (rapid tranquillisation).

Sedation and tranquillisation
■ Tranquillisation is related to DA receptor-blocking action.
■ Sedation is related to the antihistamine action and the α-adrenergic blocking properties (phenothiazines are therefore very sedative).

Antipsychotic action
The reduction of acute, positive schizophreniform symptoms (i.e. hallucinations, delusions, some aspects of thought disorder) is related to DA receptor-blocking action.

Some relevant clinical findings in acute treatment
■ In the 1964 National Institutes of Mental Health study, 463 patients with acute schizophrenia were each given a six-week trial of either chlorpromazine, fluphenazine, thioridazine or placebo. 75% of the patients improved on antipsychotics compared with 25% on placebo.
■ Antipsychotics alone are as good as antipsychotics plus psychotherapy. Both are better than psychotherapy alone or milieu therapy. ECT is better than psychotherapy but not as good as antipsychotics (NB: not recommended by NICE in the UK, see Chapter 4).
■ A meta-analysis of placebo-controlled trials with chlorpromazine showed it was better than placebo in all 26 studies at doses over 400–500 mg per day.

Relapse prevention
Antipsychotics also protect against relapse of positive symptoms.

■ When patients stable on depot were transferred to either fluphenazine or placebo for nine months, 8% of patients on fluphenazine relapsed compared with 66% on placebo.

- In a review of 66 studies (covering 1958–93), with follow-up of about eight months, the relapse rate in the medication withdrawal groups was 53% compared with 16% in the maintenance groups.
- In a review of 22 patient cohorts comparing gradual with abrupt discontinuation of medication, abrupt discontinuation resulted in a cumulative relapse rate of about 46% at six months and 56% at 24 months; gradual reduction halved the six-month relapse rate.

Adverse effects of antipsychotic drugs

Extrapyramidal side-effects (EPSE)

Motor side-effects are generated by the blockade of DA receptors in the basal ganglia (see Chapter 1). They are now more rarely seen in patients treated with the newer atypical antipsychotics but may be seen when higher doses are used. There are four main forms (Table 3.4).

Table 3.4 *Extrapyramidal side-effects*

1. Acute dystonia	Oculogyric crisis
	Torticollis
	Tongue protrusion
	Facial grimacing
2. Pseudo-parkinsonism	Muscular rigidity
	Resting tremor
	Akinesia
3. Akathisia	
4. Tardive syndromes	Dyskinesia
	Dystonia
	Akathisia

Acute dystonia and pseudo-parkinsonism

- These effects are more likely with antipsychotics, which have no intrinsic anticholinergic action (e.g. butyrophenones), and are less likely with antipsychotics with intrinsic anticholinergic properties (e.g. phenothiazines). This is because of the reciprocal actions of DA and cholinergic systems in the basal ganglia. These side-effects, by definition, are also less likely with atypical antipsychotics.
- Treatment of EPSE:
  - Reduce dose.

- Change drug to atypical antipsychotic.
- Anticholinergic medication, e.g. procyclidine or trihexyphenidyl (benzhexol). These drugs should not be coprescribed with antipsychotics routinely (i.e. in the absence of EPSE) as there is potential for abuse and they may retard antipsychotic effects. Some studies suggest that up 80% of patients chronically treated with anticholinergics can have the medication withdrawn without adverse effect.
- DA agonists (e.g. bromocriptine) may be used to treat persistent rigidity/akinesia. There is, however, a theoretical risk of aggravation of psychosis symptoms.

Akathisia
- A highly unpleasant physical and psychological restlessness.
- The precise cause is unknown and it is difficult to treat:
  - The simplest strategy is dose reduction – anticholinergics do not appear to confer benefit.
  - Diazepam and β-blockers may be helpful.

Tardive syndromes
- These are serious, disfiguring and often permanent movement disorders.
- The most common manifestation is tardive dyskinesia (Table 3.5) but dystonia and akathisia may also be present or predominate. Most commonly causes involuntary movement of the mouth or tongue though any muscle groups may be affected.
- The mechanism by which tardive dyskinesia occurs is poorly understood. Most theories focus on the disruption of D_1/D_2 receptor stimulation balance by antipsychotics but significant incidence of dyskinesia has also been observed in untreated schizophrenic patients.
- The disorder affects about 40–50% of long-term-treated patients usually coming on after months to years of treatment (hence tardive), but cases have been reported after a single episode of exposure to an antipsychotic. The incidence is highest in the first few years of treatment, with men and women equally affected.
- The risk of tardive dyskinesia increases with age, and may occur in normal ageing without antipsychotic exposure. The emergence of tardive dyskinesia is not predicted by the dose of antipsychotic used, or whether anticholinergic medication has been employed.
- Treatment of tardive dyskinesia:
  - If possible, the antipsychotic (and any associated anticholinergic) med-

ication should be gradually withdrawn or reduced: an initial exacerbation of the dyskinesia can be expected.

– Consider clozapine as an alternative antipsychotic.
– Consider benzodiazepines (e.g. clonazepam).
– Consider tetrabenazine (a vesicular DA depleter).
– There are open trials of many drugs (e.g. vitamin E) but controlled data are lacking.
– Neurosurgery (pallidotomy) may be helpful in extreme cases.
– Up to approximately 55% of patients may show recovery within a year with antipsychotic reduction.

Table 3.5 *Signs of tardive dyskinesia*

Ocular muscles	**Neck**
Blinking	Retrocollis
Blepharospasm	Torticollis
Facial	**Trunk**
Spasms	Shoulder shrugging
Tics	Pelvis rotation or thrusting
Grimaces	Diaphragmatic jerks
	Rocking
Oral	Forced retroflexion
Pouting	
Sucking	**Limbs**
Lip smacking	Finger movements
Pursing	Wrist torsion and flexion
	Arm writhing or ballismus
Masticatory	Ankle torsion and flexion
Chewing	Foot tapping
Lateral movements	Toe movements
Lingual	**Others**
Tongue protrusion	Generalised rigidity
'Fly-catching' tongue	
Writhing movements	
Pharyngeal	
Palatal movements	
Swallowing	
Abnormal sounds	

Neuroleptic malignant syndrome (NMS)

■ A relatively rare (0.5–1% of patients) but severe syndrome characterised by:
  – muscular rigidity;
  – decreased conscious level;
  – hyperthermia;
  – labile blood pressure;
  – increased creatine kinase.
■ The disorder evolves rapidly over 24–72 hours and lasts for 10–14 days if untreated. Between 5–20% of patients on oral medication and up to 30% of patients on depot formulations who develop the syndrome will die from the condition if untreated. The usual cause of death is renal failure secondary to rhabdomyolysis.

Treatment of neuroleptic malignant syndrome
■ The syndrome represents a serious medical emergency.
  – Antipsychotic drugs must be withdrawn immediately.
  – Dantroline may be used to reduce muscle spasm.
  – The DA agonist bromocriptine may be employed to reverse anti-dopaminergic effects.
  – ECT, which activates DA systems, has also been used.
  – Intensive care facilities may be required.
■ If it is necessary to use antipsychotic medication after recovery, a two-week interval should be observed and a structurally dissimilar antipsychotic gradually introduced with careful monitoring.

Other effects of antipsychotics

See Table 3.6.

Table 3.6 *Other possible effects of antipsychotics*

Effect	
Anticholinergic:	Dry mouth Constipation Blurred vision
Anti-adrenergic:	Postural hypotension
Cardiotoxicity:	Slowing of cardiac conduction time (increased QTc) leading to sudden death (especially thioridazine, pimozide) ? Alleged myocarditis
Hepatotoxicity:	Chronically raised liver enzymes
Impaired glucose tolerance/ diabetes mellitus:	Clozapine, other atypicals (NB increased baseline risk in schizophrenia)
Weight gain:	Especially clozapine, olanzapine, chlorpromazine
Blood dyscrasias:	Well known with clozapine but shared by all antipsychotics to a lesser extent
Photosensitivity:	(Especially chlorpromazine) use sun block

Atypical antipsychotics

Definitions of atypicality

■ A number of factors have been proposed as involved in defining atypicality:
  - ↑efficacy for positive symptoms;
  - ↑efficacy for negative symptoms;
  - ↓tendency to cause EPSE;
  - failure to ↑prolactin.

■ However, the most parsimonious definitions are related to tendency to cause EPSE:
  - preclinically – an effective antipsychotic that does not produce catalepsy in rats; or
  - clinically – a drug with wide therapeutic ratio for antipsychotic effects and EPSE such that EPSE are not seen at clinically effective doses.

Mechanisms of atypicality

Atypical antipsychotics vary in their pharmacological properties. It is likely that a number of mechanisms confer different aspects of atypical status.

- Reduced EPSE:
  - $\downarrow D_2$ antagonism;
  - high 5-HT_2:D_2 binding ratio;
  - limbic selective D_2 antagonism;
  - 'loose binding' to dopamine D_2-like receptors;
  - D_2 receptor partial agonism;
  - cholinergic M_1 receptor antagonism (NB high levels of M_1 antagonism may exacerbate psychosis).
- Reduced hyperprolactinaemia:
  - $\downarrow D_2$ antagonism;
  - D_2 receptor partial agonism.
- Increased efficacy against positive symptoms. Proposed mechanisms include:
  - differential D_1 binding;
  - high 5-HT_2: D_2 ratio;
  - high D_4 binding;
  - other relative binding/activity ratios.
- Increased efficacy against negative symptoms. Proposed mechanisms include:
  - pre- versus postsynaptic D_2 antagonism;
  - 5-HT_2 antagonism;
  - D_2 receptor partial agonism;
  - absence of EPSE may simulate an effect on negative symptoms.

Clozapine represents the prototypical atypical antipsychotic, illustrating the features described above:

- Low incidence of EPSE.
- Does not stimulate prolactin secretion.
- Effective in treatment-resistant cases.
- Improves negative as well as positive symptoms.
- Receptor binding affinity profile: $H_1 > M_1 = \alpha_1 > 5\text{-}HT_2 > D_2 = D_1 = \alpha_2$.
- Relatively low affinity for D_2 receptor.
- D_2 limbic selectivity.

Distribution of pharmacological mechanisms amongst atypical drugs

- High affinity for cholinergic M_1 receptors: thioridazine, clozapine.
- Low affinity for striatal D_2 receptors: clozapine, quetiapine, olanzapine.

- Higher affinity for 5-HT$_{2A}$ receptors than for striatal D$_2$ receptors: risperidone, sertindole, ziprasidone, olanzapine, clozapine, quetiapine.
- Higher affinity for limbic D$_2$ and D$_2$-like receptors than for striatal D$_2$ receptors: clozapine, sertindole, amisulpiride, quetiapine, risperidone (limbic selectivity is lost at higher doses for all, except possibly clozapine).
- 'Loose binding' to striatal D$_2$-like receptors: clozapine, quetiapine, ?risperidone, ?sertindole, ?olanzapine (but may be a pharmacokinetic rather than pharmacodynamic effect).
- D$_2$ receptor partial agonism: aripiprazole.

Individual atypical antipsychotics (listed alphabetically)

Currently, amisulpiride, aripiprazole, olanzapine, quetiapine, risperidone, sertindole (with restrictions) and zotepine are licensed in the UK.

Amisulpride

Pharmacology
- selective and equipotent antagonism for D$_2$ and D$_3$;
- limbic selective;
- negligible affinity for other receptors.

Efficacy
- As efficacious as haloperidol for acute and chronic schizophrenia.
- Optimum dose 400–800 mg per day.
- At 50–300 mg effective for patients with mainly negative symptoms.

Side-effects
- Low EPSE similar to placebo at lower doses.
- Less weight gain compared with risperidone or olanzapine.
- Dose-dependent EPSE and prolactinaemia at higher doses.

Aripiprazole

Pharmacology
- D$_2$ receptor partial agonist;
- partial agonist at 5-HT$_{1A}$ receptors;
- high-affinity antagonist at 5-HT$_{2A}$ receptors;
- low/moderate affinity antagonist at H$_1$ and α_1 receptors;
- no anticholinergic effect.

Efficacy
- ■ As effective as haloperidol and olanzapine for acute and chronic schizophrenia.
- ■ Optimum dose 15 mg per day, (maximum 30 mg).
- ■ Effective in the acute treatment of mania.

Side-effects
- ■ Low EPSE similar to placebo at all doses (initial akathisia can occur in approx. the first two weeks of treatment).
- ■ Does not increase plasma prolactin levels (and may decrease them).
- ■ Less weight gain than olanzapine.

Olanzapine
Pharmacology
- ■ related to clozapine;
- ■ receptor antagonism: $5\text{-HT}_2 = H_1 = M_1 > D_2 > \alpha_1 > D_1$;
- ■ some D_2 limbic selectivity.

Efficacy
- ■ As effective as haloperidol for positive symptoms of schizophrenia.
- ■ Some evidence of better efficacy against negative symptoms of schizophrenia.
- ■ Better than risperidone for mood symptoms.
- ■ Effective in the acute treatment of mania and maintenance treatment of bipolar disorder.

Side-effects
- ■ EPSE similar to placebo in clinical doses;
- ■ sedation;
- ■ weight gain;
- ■ dizziness;
- ■ dry mouth;
- ■ constipation;
- ■ less increase in prolactin than haloperidol or risperidone.

Quetiapine
Pharmacology
- ■ receptor antagonism: $H_1 > \alpha_1 > 5\text{-HT}_2 > \alpha_2 > D_2$;
- ■ D_2 limbic selectivity.

Efficacy
- As effective as haloperidol and chlorpromazine for schizophrenia.
- Possible efficacy for negative symptoms.
- Effective in the acute treatment of mania.

Side-effects
- EPSE = placebo;
- no increase in prolactin;
- sedation;
- dizziness;
- constipation;
- infrequent – dry mouth, weight gain.

Risperidone

Pharmacology
- receptor antagonism: $5\text{-HT}_2 > D_2 = \alpha_1 = \alpha_2$;
- little histamine H_1 affinity;
- minimal D_1, 5-HT_1 affinity;
- D_2 limbic selective only at lower doses.

Efficacy
- 11+ multicentre double-blind trials in schizophrenia;
- possible bell-shaped dose response curve;
- uncertain if effective for negative symptoms;
- effective in the acute treatment of mania.

Side-effects
- markedly less pseudoparkinsonism than typical antipsychotics at lower doses, but dystonias and akathisia can occur;
- tachycardia;
- some weight gain;
- fewer treatment dropouts than with typical antipsychotics.

Sertindole

Withdrawn due to concerns about ↑QTc. Limited reintroduction in 2002 in Europe under strict monitoring

Pharmacology
- D_2, 5-HT_2 and α_1 antagonist;
- D_2 limbic selectivity.

Efficacy
- ■ Effective against positive and negative symptoms of schizophrenia.

Side-effects
- ■ EPSE = placebo.
- ■ Minimal short-term ↑prolactin.
- ■ ↑QTc – needs ECG monitoring.
- ■ Nasal congestion, decreased ejaculatory volume, postural hypotension and dry mouth.
- ■ Occasionally raised liver enzymes.

Ziprasidone
Licensed in the USA and parts of Europe; not in the UK.

Pharmacology
- ■ receptor antagonism: $5\text{-}HT_{2A} > D_2 > 5\text{-}HT_{1A} > \alpha_1 > H_1$.
- ■ ?Limbic selective D_2.
- ■ No anticholinergic effect.
- ■ Weak 5-HT and NA re-uptake inhibition.

Efficacy
- ■ Perhaps slightly more effective than haloperidol.
- ■ Possible efficacy for negative symptoms of schizophrenia.
- ■ Possible efficacy for depressive symptoms in schizophrenia.
- ■ Effective in the acute treatment of mania.

Side-effects
- ■ EPSE = placebo.
- ■ No appreciable weight gain.
- ■ No appreciable cholinergic side-effects.
- ■ Insomnia, pharyngitis, rash and tremor more common than with placebo.
- ■ Concerns over tendency to ↑QTc.
- ■ Appears to *reduce* prolactin relative to placebo.
- ■ Headache, nausea and insomnia most common side-effects (but occur in <10% of patients).

Zotepine
Pharmacology
- ■ High affinity for D_1 and D_2 receptors, also $5\text{-}HT_2$, $5\text{-}HT_6$ and $5\text{-}HT_7$ receptors.
- ■ Inhibits NA re-uptake.

Efficacy

■ Effective against positive and negative symptoms of schizophrenia but controlled trial data limited.

Side-effects

■ EPSE less than typical antipsychotics;

■ seizures at higher doses (above 300 mg);

■ weight gain;

■ sedation;

■ constipation, asthenia, dry mouth, akathisia;

■ raised hepatic enzymes.

References

Key references

Bollini P, Pampallona S, Orza MJ et al. Antipsychotic drugs: is more worse? A meta-analysis of the published randomised controlled trials. Psychol Med 1994; 24:307–16

Creese I, Burt DR, Snyder SH. Dopamine receptor binding predicts clinical and pharmacological potencies of antischizophrenic drugs. Science 1976; 192:481–3

Cunningham-Owens DG. Adverse effects of antipsychotic agents. Do newer agents offer advantages? Drugs 1996; 51(6):895–930.

Geddes J, Freemantle N, Harrison P, Bebbington P. Atypical antipsychotics in the treatment of schizophrenia: systematic overview and meta-regression analysis. BMJ 2000; 321:1371–6

Hirsch S, Gaind R, Rohde PD et al. Outpatient maintenance of chronic schizophrenia patients with long-acting fluphenazine: double-blind placebo trial. BMJ 1973; 1:633–7

Johnstone E, Crow TJ, Frith CD et al. Mechanism of the antipsychotic effect in the treatment of schizophrenia. Lancet 1978; i:848–51

Johnstone EC, Crow TJ, Frith CD, Owens DG. The Northwick Park 'functional' psychosis study: diagnosis and treatment response. Lancet 1988; 2(8603):119–25

Kane J, Honigfeld G, Singer J, Meltzer H. Clozapine for the treatment-resistant schizophrenic: a double-blind comparison with chlorpromazine. Arch Gen Psychiatry 1988; 45:789–96

Viguera AC, Baldessarini RJ, Hegarty JD et al. Clinical risk following abrupt and gradual withdrawal of maintenance neuroleptic treatment. Arch Gen Psychiatry 1997; 54:49–55

Wyatt RJ. Neuroleptics and the natural course of schizophrenia. Schizophr Bull 1991; 17:325–51

Further reading

Busatto GF, Kerwin RW. Perspectives on the role of serotonergic mechanisms in the pharmacology of schizophrenia. J Psychopharmacol 1997; 11(1):3–12

Carpenter WT, Jr. Maintenence therapy of persons with schizophrenia. J Clin Psychiatry 1996; 57(Suppl. 9):10–18 (NB This whole supplement is good)

Davis JM, Andriukaitis S. The natural course of schizophrenia and effective maintainence treatment. J Clin Psychopharmacol 1986; 6(Suppl. 1):2–10

Gilbert PL, Harris J, McAdams LA, Jeste DV. Neuroleptic withdrawal in schizophrenic patients. Arch Gen Psychiatry 1995; 52:173–88

Hegarty JD, Baldessarini RJ, Tohen M *et al*. One hundred years of schizophrenia: meta-analysis of the outcome literature. Am J Psychiatry 1994; 151:1409–16

Kuperberg G, Kerwin R, Murray R. Developments in the pharmacological treatment of schizophrenia. Expert Opinion on Investigational Drugs 2002; 11(10):1335–41

Laruelle M, Abi-Dargham A, van Dick *et al*. Single photon emission computerized tomography imaging of amphetamine-induced dopamine release in drug-free schizophrenic subjects. Proc Natl Acad Sci USA 1996; 93:9235–40

Laruelle M, Abi-Dargham A, Gil R *et al*. Increased dopamine transmission in schizophrenia: relationship to illness phases. Biol Psychiatry 1999; 46:56–72

Malhotra AK, Litman RE, Pickar D. Adverse effects of antipsychotics drugs. Drug Safety 1993; 9:429–36

McGurk SR, Meltzer HY. The effects of atypical antipsychotic drugs on cognitive functioning in schizophrenia. Schizophr Res 1999; 25:233–55

National Institute for Clinical Excellence Clinical Guideline 1. Schizophrenia: Core interventions in the treatment and management of schizophrenia in primary and secondary care, 2002. http://www.nice.org.uk

National Institute for Clinical Excellence Technology Appraisal No. 43. Guidance on the use of newer (atypical) antipsychotic drugs for the treatment of schizophrenia, 2002. http://www.nice.org.uk

Seeman P, Guan HC, van Tol HH. Dopamine D_4 receptor elevated in schizophrenia. Nature 1993; 365:441–5

Seeman P. Atypical antipsychotics: mechanism of action. Can J Psychiatry 2002; 47(1):27–38

Staddon S, Arranz MJ, Mancama D *et al*. Clinical applications of pharmacogenetics in psychiatry. Psychopharmacology 2002; 162(1):18–23.

Stahl S. Essential Psychopharmacology: Neuroscientific Basis and Practical Implications, 2nd edn. Cambridge, UK: Cambridge University Press, 2000

Taylor D. Low-dose typical antipsychotics – a brief evaluation. Psychiatr Bull 2000; 24:465–8

Taylor D, Paton C, Kerwin RW. The South London and Maudsley NHS Trust 2003 Prescribing Guidelines, 7th edn. London: Martin Dunitz, 2003

Travis MJ. Schizophrenia and other psychotic disorders: therapeutic armamentarium. In: Biological Psychiatry (D'haenen H, den Boer JA, Willner P, eds). London: John Wiley, pp 685–700; 2003

4 Antidepressants and electroconvulsive therapy

History

The first effective antidepressant agents of the modern era were discovered by chance in the late 1950s:

- Iproniazid (monoamine oxidase inhibitor, MAOI): developed originally as an antitubercular drug.
- Imipramine (tricyclic): developed originally as a chlorpromazine analogue (1957).
- MAOIs and tricyclics have the common property of interacting with monoamine systems (DA, NA, 5-HT).

The monoamine hypothesis of depression

The monoamine hypothesis was originally proposed in the 1960s based on the actions of drugs (reserpine observed to cause depression and antidepressants to relieve depression).

- Schildkraut – proposed catecholamines (NA, DA) to be functionally deficient in depression and elevated in activity in mania.
- Ashcroft – proposed indolamines (5-HT) to be functionally deficient in depression. This led to the development of 5-HT-selective drugs in the 1970s resulting in the selective serotonin re-uptake inhibitors (SSRIs).
- It has been much modified over succeeding decades, with the focus moving from neurotransmitter turnover, through receptor regulation, to intracellular changes.

■ A current formulation proposes that a common mechanism of antidepressant action is to increase 5-HT neurotransmission by altering receptor sensitivity.

■ For example, chronic 5-HT re-uptake blockade with SSRIs results in down-regulation of 5-HT$_{1A}$ receptors on the cell bodies of serotonergic neurones in the brain stem, thus disabling negative feedback, restoring cell firing rate resulting in increased synaptic 5-HT (Fig. 4.1).

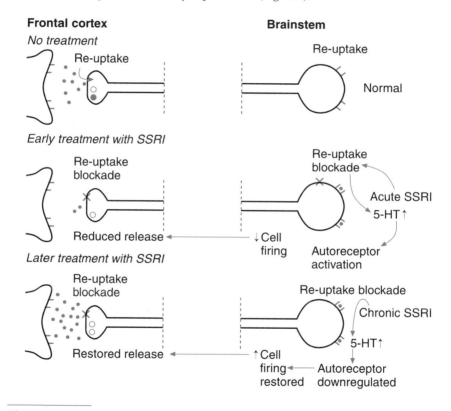

Figure 4.1 *Current 5-HT hypothesis of how antidepressant drugs work.*

■ The hypothesis does not explain satisfactorily the similarity in efficacy of very different agents acting differentially on monoamine systems.

Furthermore, evidence for primary monoamine disturbance in depressed subjects is limited and inconsistent.

Evidence for the role of serotonin, dopamine and noradrenaline in the aetiology of major depression

The action of antidepressants on monoamine neurotransmission does not by itself mean that these systems are abnormal in depression. The main evidence is summarised below.

Serotonin (5-HT)

- Reduced 5-HT metabolites in the cerebrospinal fluid of sufferers, and in brain tissue post-mortem.
- Increased platelet/brain 5-HT$_2$ receptors.
- Downregulation/reduced numbers of postsynaptic 5-HT$_{1A}$ receptors (neuroendocrine studies: prolactin response to tryptophan infusion; buspirone-induced hypothermia; positron emission tomography (PET) studies of brain 5-HT$_{1A}$ receptor binding).
- Relapse of depression induced by tryptophan depletion in SSRI-treated and drug-free recovered depressed patients.

Noradrenaline (NA)

- Reduced levels of the NA metabolite MHPG in the urine of depressed subjects.
- Possible postsynaptic α_2 downregulation (neuroendocrine studies: abnormal growth hormone response to clonidine; insulin-induced hypoglycaemia).
- Decreased responses to β-receptor agonists in depression.
- Relapse of depression induced by α-methyl paratyrosine (NA synthesis inhibitor) in patients treated with NA re-uptake inhibitors.

Dopamine (DA)

- Increased D$_2$ receptor numbers in some PET studies of depressed patients.
- Mood elevating effects of DA-releasing psychostimulants.
- Possible antipsychotic-induced depression (high dose – postsynaptic DA receptor blockade).
- Possible antipsychotic antidepressant activity (low dose – presynaptic DA autoreceptor blockade).
- Preclinical studies consistently implicate DA systems in neural basis of reward (related to anhedonia).

The role of the HPA axis

Abnormalities in the regulation of the hypothalmic–pituitary–adrenal (HPA) axis, though neither specific to depressive disorder, nor demonstrable in every case, are implicated in the aetiology of depressive disorder.

■ Many depressed patients exhibit elevated cortisol levels and an insensitivity to dexamethasone-induced cortisol suppression.

■ Complex interactions between 5-HT and corticosteroid systems in the central nervous system (CNS) are only now beginning to be understood, and may account for some of the relationships between the effects of stress, mood dysregulation and cognitive dysfunction encountered in depressive disorder.

■ The toxic effects of cortisol dysregulation may account for the evidence of degenerative changes seen in the brain in depressive disorder.

■ Adverse early experience – physical, emotional, or sexual abuse – may alter HPA axis function in a lasting way, conferring vulnerability to depression and stress-related disorders in adulthood.

■ Recent trials suggest that glucocorticoid receptor antagonists, such as mifepristone, may be effective treatments in severe depressive disorder. Similarly, the activities of hormones which regulate the HPA axis, such as corticotrophin-releasing hormone, and other agents active at the various glucocorticoid and mineralocorticoid receptors in the brain, are attracting interest as potential targets for future antidepressant design.

The neurotrophic and neuroplasticity hypotheses

■ Recent research indicates that in chronic severe depressive disorders alterations in brain structure may occur, particularly frontal and temporal cortical atrophy, possibly mediated by corticosteroid abnormalities.

■ Intriguingly, antidepressant agents (including electroconvulsive stimulation, ECS) have common cellular effects leading to enhanced expression of neuroprotective proteins that bolster neuronal survival and regulate synaptic connectivity.

  – In rats, antidepressant drugs and ECS promote enhanced cell production in the dentate gyrus of the hippocampus. These effects may act to reverse the proposed toxic effects of HPA axis abnormalities (Fig. 4.2).

  – Preliminary studies in some stress-related disorders, such as post-traumatic stress disorder, suggest that antidepressant drugs can reverse volumetric abnormalities in limbic system structures, such as the hippocampus.

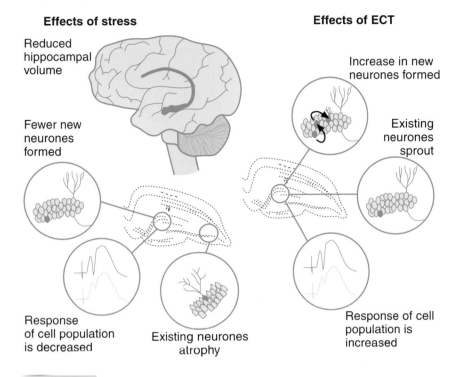

Effects of stress

Reduced hippocampal volume

Fewer new neurones formed

Response of cell population is decreased

Existing neurones atrophy

Effects of ECT

Increase in new neurones formed

Existing neurones sprout

Response of cell population is increased

Figure 4.2 *Reciprocal effects of stress and ECT on neurones (Courtesy of Dr CA Stewart, University of Dundee).*

Antidepressant drugs

Most antidepressants have acute effects on monoamine neurotransmission (Fig. 4.3).

Tricyclic antidepressants (TCAs)

Neurochemical effects: spectrum of activity

- 5-HT re-uptake inhibition.
- NA re-uptake inhibition.
- Tertiary amines are generally more potent at blocking 5-HT uptake.
- Secondary amines more potent at blocking NA uptake.
- Anticholinergic effects.
- Antihistaminergic effects

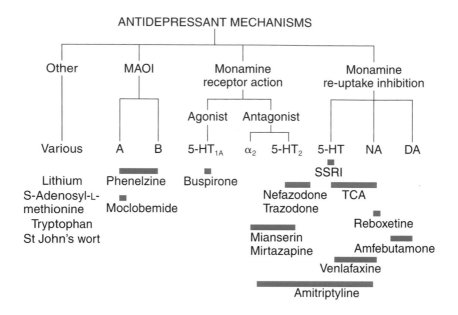

Figure 4.3 *Acute pharmacology of some antidepressants.*

Pharmacokinetics

■ Rapidly absorbed, widely distributed.

■ Genetic variation in liver metabolism.

■ Tertiary amines metabolised to secondary amines, e.g. amitriptyline to nortriptyline; imipramine to desmethylimipramine.

■ Comparative pharmacology of TCAs is shown in Table 4.1.

Table 4.1 *Selective comparative pharmacology of TCAs*

	$t_{1/2}$ (h) (active metabolite)	NA uptake inhibition	5-HT uptake inhibition	Anti-cholinergic	Sedation
Amitriptyline	16 (36)	++	+++	+++	+++
Imipramine	16 (24)	++	+++	++	++
Clomipramine	18 (36)	+	+++	++	+
Nortriptyline	36	+++	+	++	+
Dosulepin (dothiepin)	20 (40)	+	+	++	++
Lofepramine	5 (24)	+++	+	+	+

Efficacy

- Acute treatment of episode of depression: 55–70% response rate, 10–20 day delay.
- Effective in relapse prevention.
- Need adequate dose (125–150 mg imipramine or equivalent) – requires dose titration (inconvenient for doctor and patient).
- Useful in adults, agitation, retardation, severe – may be more effective in severe depression in inpatients compared to SSRIs.
- Less useful in the elderly, psychotic, physically ill, those with a history of bipolar disorder and the suicidal.

Side-effects

- *Anticholinergic*: Dry mouth, constipation, urinary retention, accommodation problems, glaucoma.
- *Antihistaminergic*: Sedation, weight gain.
- *α-Noradrenergic blockade*: Postural hypotension, sedation.
- *5-HT$_2$ blockade*: weight gain (amitriptyline).
- *Cardiotoxic*: QT prolongation, ST elevation, AV block, membrane stabilisation, arrhythmias.
- *Neurotoxic*: Delirium, movement disorders, convulsions.
- *Discontinuation syndrome* (see also SSRIs below): General somatic symptoms, insomnia, vivid dreams, gastrointestinal symptoms, mood symptoms including anxiety, agitation, rarely psychosis.
- *Manic switch in bipolar patients.*

Contraindications

- Heart block.
- Hypomania or mania.
- Recent myocardial infarction.

Interactions

Useful interactions (with caution):
- SSRIs, lithium, L-tryptophan.

Problematic interactions:

- MAOIs (especially clomipramine and tranylcypromine).
- Antiepileptics (barbiturates decrease TCA levels).
- Cimetidine increases TCA levels.
- Warfarin action potentiated.
- Alcohol potentiates TCA sedation.

Selective serotonin re-uptake inhibitors (SSRIs)

Increasingly, SSRIs are the first-line treatment for depression.

Neurochemistry

All share the property of relatively selective 5-HT re-uptake blockade but are structurally distinct, and each has other actions on different neurotransmitter systems, some of which may be undocumented.

Pharmacokinetics

- Rapidly absorbed.
- Hepatic metabolism.
- Some have active metabolites (Table 4.2).
- Variation in cytochrome P450 inhibition and potential for drug interactions (see Table 4.2).
- Low concentrations in breast milk (highest fluoxetine).
- Withdrawal effects possible with short half-life drugs (paroxetine greatest, fluoxetine least).

Table 4.2 *Selective comparative pharmacology of SSRIs*

	Active metabolite	$t_{1/2}$ (h) (active metabolite)	Cytochrome P450 inhibition
Citalopram	–	36	–
Escitalopram (S-enantiomer of citalopram)	–	36	–
Fluoxetine	+++	72 (200)	+++ (2D6, 3A4, 2C19)
Fluvoxamine	–	15	++ (1A2, 2C19)
Paroxetine	–	20	+++ (2D6, 2C9)
Sertraline	+	25 (66)	+ (2D6)

Efficacy

- Acute treatment of episode of depression: 55–70% response rate.
- 10–20 day delay in response.
- Effective in relapse prevention.
- Little evidence of dose-response in usual dose range: less need for dose titration.
- Useful in the elderly, depression with anxiety/OCD, suicidal patients (safer in overdose than tricyclics).

- Recent evidence that escitalopram may be more effective, or have an earlier onset of action, than citalopram and have equal efficacy to venlafaxine. This is attributed to escitalopram binding to both the re-uptake site and an allosteric site causing conformational change in the 5-HT transporter and enhancing re-uptake blockade. R-enantiomer blocks this effect. This is not seen with other SSRIs. These are mostly company data so claims need independent verification.

Side-effects

- Nausea/vomiting (activation of postsynaptic 5-HT$_3$ receptors).
- Agitation.
- Akathisia.
- Parkinsonism (uncommon).
- Sedation/dizziness (10–20%).
- Convulsions (rare).
- Sexual dysfunction common in males and females (possibly activation of postsynaptic 5-HT$_2$ receptors). Appears most prominent with paroxetine, possibly least with fluvoxamine.
- Controversial: increased risk of suicidality which may be due to agitation/akathisia. See also Chapter 8. In the UK an expert group was set up in 2003 by the Medicines and Healthcare products Regulatory Authority (MHRA) to investigate this possible side-effect.
- Discontinuation syndrome related to half-life (especially paroxetine, rare with fluoxetine) (see below).

Interactions

Useful interactions (with caution):

- TCAs, lithium (possible serotonin syndrome).

Problematic interactions:

- MAOIs (toxicity, serotonin syndrome).
- L-Tryptophan.
- With fluvoxamine (due to cytochrome P450-1A2 inhibition): caffeine, clozapine, theophylline.
- With fluoxetine and paroxetine (due to cytochrome P450-2D6, -3A3/4 inhibition): antipsychotics, opiates, TCAs.
- St John's wort (serotonin syndrome).

Serotonin syndrome

Acute toxic syndrome due to increased 5-HT activity (can be confused with neuroleptic malignant syndrome, NMS, see Chapter 3).

- Confusion.
- Myoclonic jerks, hyperreflexia.
- Pyrexia, sweating, autonomic instability (usually less than in NMS).
- Gastrointestinal symptoms.
- Mood change, mania.

SSRI discontinuation syndrome

- Sensory abnormalities (including electric shock-like sensations).
- Dysequilibrium (dizziness, etc.).
- Insomnia, increased dreams.
- General somatic symptoms (headache, lethargy, etc.).
- Gastrointestinal symptoms.
- Mood change (depression, anxiety/agitation, rarely mania).
- Psychosis (rarely).

Monoamine oxidase inhibitors (MAOIs)

Neurochemistry

Inhibition of MAO enzymes A and B:

- MAO present in periphery, especially the gut, as well as the CNS.
- MAO-A metabolises NA, 5-HT and tyramine.
- MAO-B metabolises DA, tyramine and phenylethylamine.
- MAOIs increases the storage and release of 5-HT and NA.
- Traditional MAOIs (phenelzine, tranylcypromine): irreversible inhibition.
- Moclobemide: Reversible Inhibitor of MAO-A (RIMA), potential for interaction with indirect sympathomimetics greatly reduced as drug displaced from enzyme.

Pharmacokinetics

- Rapid absorption.
- Toxic levels can occur in slow acetylators.
- Half-life not as important as the time taken to replace stores of MAO after irreversible blockade (two weeks).

Efficacy

Traditional MAOIs are third-line treatment but retain important place in therapy. Useful in:

■ severe depression, especially with lethargy and poor motivation;
■ treatment resistance: may also be combined with lithium and/or L-tryptophan;
■ anxiety states/OCD;
■ atypical depression – depression with mood reactivity, excessive sleeping and weight gain, sensitivity to rejection.

Side-effects
■ Postural hypotension.
■ Restlessness, insomnia.
■ Peripheral oedema – beware ascites/pleural effusion.
■ Nausea, dizziness, sexual difficulties, sweating, tremor.

Interactions
Hypertensive crisis occurs with tyramine-containing foods and some drugs (dietary tyramine is normally inactivated in the gut by MAO). Moclobemide has very limited potential for this interaction.

Hypertensive reaction
■ Symptoms:
    – Flushing.
    – Headache.
    – Increased blood pressure.
    – Rarely cerebrovascular accident.
■ Causes:
    – Tyramine-containing foods, e.g. cheese, yeast extracts, hung game, some alcoholic drinks, broad bean pods, pickled herring.
    – Sympathomimetics drugs (e.g. non-prescription cold remedies).
■ Management:
    – Prevention: education, food warning leaflets.
    – Treatment of hypertensive crisis: α-blockade with phentolamine or chlorpromazine.

Other drug interactions
■ Other antidepressants – excitement and hyperpyrexia.
■ Pethidine – respiratory depression, coma.
■ Alcohol, barbiturates – CNS depression.
■ Insulin – impaired blood glucose control.

Contraindications

- Cardiovascular disease.
- Cerebrovascular disease.
- Children.
- Epilepsy.
- Hepatic disease.
- Phaeochromocytoma.
- Hyperthyroidism (tranylcypromine).

Notes on other antidepressants

Phenylpiperazines

E.g. trazodone, nefazodone.

- Relatively weak serotonin re-uptake inhibition.
- $5\text{-}HT_2$ antagonist properties, which may have antidepressant and anxiolytic properties, as well as reducing the impact of serotonin re-uptake on sexual function.
- Relatively safe in overdose.
- Trazodone is somewhat sedative.
- Nefazodone withdrawn from European market in 2003 due to hepatotoxicity.

Noradrenaline re-uptake inhibitors (NARI)

E.g. reboxetine.

- Relatively specific re-uptake inhibitor of noradrenaline. May have alerting properties.

Serotonin and noradrenaline re-uptake inhibitors (SNRI)

Also known as 'dual action' re-uptake inhibitors, e.g. venlafaxine, milnacipran (available in France and Japan) and duloxetine (due to be marketed in 2004/5).

Venlafaxine

- Selective 5-HT and NA uptake inhibitor (a 'clean' tricyclic?).
- NA re-uptake inhibition only evident at higher doses.
- May have more rapid onset of action and enhanced efficacy in severe depressive disorder.
- Blood pressure needs to be monitored when dose exceeds 200 mg daily.

L-Tryptophan

- Precursor of 5-HT.
- Weak antidepressant, adjunct for MAOIs and TCAs.
- Some sedation, watch for eosinophilia myalgia syndrome, myoclonus and serotonergic syndrome.
- Currently only available on 'named patient' basis in the UK.

a$_2$ Adrenoceptor antagonists

E.g. mirtazapine, mianserin.

Mirtazapine

- Also known as a noradrenaline- and serotonin-specific antidepressant (NaSSa).
- 5-HT$_2$, 5-HT$_3$, antihistaminergic and α_2 antagonist.
- Relatively sedative antidepressant (antihistaminergic effects), which may be less at higher doses.
- Activates NA neurones by blocking the negative feedback of NA on presynaptic α_2 receptors.
- Increased noradrenergic activity stimulates 5-HT neurone activity in the brainstem, while blockade of α_2 receptors on 5-HT terminals in the cortex enhances 5-HT release.
- Net effect is to increase activity in both NA and 5-HT systems
- Blockade of 5-HT$_2$ and 5-HT$_3$ receptors minimises sexual dysfunction and nausea.

Other putative antidepressants

- Some drugs used as mood stabilisers (see Chapter 5) also have antidepressant properties (lithium in unipolar and probably bipolar depression, lamotrigine in bipolar depression) with a lack of evidence for others even though they are commonly used first line in bipolar depression (valproate, carbamazepine).
- Atypical antipsychotics such as olanzapine may have weak antidepressant properties in bipolar depression.
- Investigational drugs include CRF antagonists (especially psychotic depression) and neurokinin$_1$ (NK$_1$) antagonists.
- St John's wort has inconsistent evidence for short-term efficacy in mild–moderate depression.

Using antidepressants effectively

- Dose (150 mg imipramine or equivalent) and duration of treatment (at least six months post remission) appear to be crucial in attaining stable remission of an acute episode.
- Even more important is effective prophylaxis, as depressive episodes are likely to be recurrent – estimated three year relapse rate following adequate treatment: placebo = 80%; 150 mg imipramine = 20%. Note that 'maintenance dose' is an obsolete concept: the dose that gets you better keeps you better!
- Antidepressant use in primary care requires special consideration: there is evidence that antidepressants may be both overprescribed (given to patients with mild disorder who are unlikely to benefit) and underprescribed (following failure to detect illness, or given in insufficient doses for inadequate periods of time).
- Meta-analyses suggest that SSRIs may be better tolerated in primary care patients, and because dose titration is less frequently necessary than with tricyclics, SSRIs are more likely to be prescribed at therapeutic doses.
- A British Association for Psychopharmacology (BAP) evidence-based guideline on the treatment of depressive disorders is available (see www.bap.org.uk), and a guideline from the National Institute for Clinical Excellence (NICE) in the UK, focusing on the treatment of depression, is expected in late 2004 (see www.nice.org.uk).

In choosing antidepressant agents consider:

- Previous response and tolerance, and patient preference.
- Tolerance and need for prophylaxis.
- Age and physical health.
- Suicidality.
- Concordance issues.
- Past history of elevated mood – tricyclics may promote 'rapid cycling' in bipolar disorder.
- Symptom profile.

Treatment-resistant depression

- Some 20–40% of patients will fail to respond to adequate doses of adequate duration of an antidepressant. In patients who do not respond at all to medication after four weeks, it is unlikely that the antidepressant will subsequently prove effective. An important exception is elderly patients, who may require longer trials.

■ Treatment-resistant depression has varying definitions but usually refers to a failure to respond to trials of two antidepressants at an adequate dose, given for an adequate period of time (greater than four weeks).

Common strategies following treatment failure include:

■ Increasing the dose of the agent.
■ Switching to another drug, often from an alternative class (though even within a class antidepressants may be chemically very different).
■ Adding lithium or triiodothyronine as adjuvent agents.
■ Combining agents (e.g. tricyclic and SSRI; venlafaxine and mirtazepine).
■ Considering electroconvulsive therapy (ECT).

The 'evidence base' is limited in this situation. With regard to augmentation therapies, the most robust evidence favours the use of lithium but this may simply reflect the limited research that this particular clinical problem has attracted to date. In any case, it is important to:

■ re-consider diagnosis;
■ appraise concordance with treatment;
■ review physical status;
■ be systematic in treatment trials.

Careful recording of the history of treatments and their outcomes and adverse events is crucial. Though beyond the scope of this chapter, consideration of specific psychological therapies, such as cognitive behavioural therapy, is essential.

Further options include:

■ Experimental strategies being investigated include the addition of atypical neuroleptics, the use of modafinil, an antinarcoleptic agent, antiglucocorticoids, newer physical treatments such as vagus nerve stimulation and transcranial magnetic stimulation.
■ Very rarely, in extreme cases, neurosurgical approaches, such as anterior cingulotomy, have been successfully used.

Electroconvulsive therapy (ECT)

Although not a psychopharmacological treatment, ECT is briefly considered because of evidence for similar effects to antidepressant drugs and its place alongside antidepressants in the treatment of severe depression.

History
- ECT has its roots in the mistaken idea that schizophrenia and epilepsy were antithetical conditions.
- Convulsions were first induced chemically.
- Later (in the 1930s) Cerletti and Binet developed the safer electrical induction of seizures. Initially, 'unmodified' ECT was used (i.e. without muscle relaxant).
- Now general anaesthesia and muscle relaxation are employed to reduce the risk of fracture during seizure activity.
- Large open trials in the 1960s and blinded, randomised placebo-controlled trials in the 1970s and 1980s demonstrated the efficacy of ECT in depressive disorder.
- It remains one of the most controversial treatments in medicine, with a poor 'media' image.
- ECT use is falling, perhaps partly as a consequence of more systematic and effective chemical and psychological treatments for depressive disorder.

Mode of action
- The mode of action of ECT, like chemical antidepressant therapy, is poorly understood.
- Similar effects on monoamine systems, as occur with chemical antidepressants, have been described; DA systems may be particularly affected.
- Perhaps counterintuitively, there is evidence that electroconvulsive stimulation has neuroprotective effects and stimulates neurogenesis in preclinical models.
- ECT is a potent anticonvulsant, and may share properties with some mood-stabilising agents effective in affective disorder.
- There is no evidence that ECT causes brain damage.

Indications
Evidence for efficacy is strongest in depressed patients with psychosis and psychomotor retardation. ECT tends to be reserved for situations where:

- alternative treatments have failed;

- a rapid response is necessary in the face of intense suicidality;
- dangerous self-neglect;
- intractable psychotic depressive states.

NICE guidance in the UK (2003, Guideline 59; see www.nice.org.uk), considering the use of ECT in depression, mania, schizophrenia and catatonia recommends that:

- its use is restricted to the short term and rapid relief of severe depression, mania or catatonia in patients who;
- have failed to respond to other treatments;
- and that it should not be used in schizophrenia or for maintenance treatment.

Procedure

- The aim of ECT is to induce safely a generalised tonic–clonic seizure lasting at least 25 seconds.
- EEG monitoring is increasingly recommended.
- Though enshrined in Royal College of Psychiatrists' guidelines, the significance of seizure length (as opposed to whether the seizure occurs at all) remains uncertain.
- The electrical stimulus is applied via two electrodes placed either bitemporally (bilateral ECT) or across one side of the head (unilateral ECT).
- Dose is measured in units of charge (amps × seconds), and the amount of charge required to induce a seizure may vary 40-fold across individuals, depending on the characteristics of the equipment used.
- Given that the intensity of side-effects induced (see below) may vary with overall electrical energy administered, many authorities advocate stimulus dosing to determine optimal parameters for individual patients.
- Some studies suggest that high-dose unilateral ECT may be as effective as bilateral ECT, but is accompanied by less cognitive dysfunction. Bifrontal electrode placement may also reduce cognitive side-effects while maintaining efficacy.
- In general, with ECT several treatments are required to achieve good outcomes, spaced by two or three days (i.e. two or three times per week). The median number of treatments given in recent audits in Scotland, England and Wales was six.
- NICE in the UK has issued a clinical guideline for the use of ECT (Guideline 59; see www.nice.org.uk). This includes recommendations for audit.
- There is considerable variation in the standards of ECT administration and the Royal College of Psychiatrists in the UK in 2003 set up an ECT accreditation service (ECTAS) to attempt to improve practice.

Clinical uses

Common

■ Depressive disorder.

■ Treatment-resistant mania.

Less common

■ Schizophrenia – may be useful in achieving symptom control in treatment-resistant schizophrenia to permit the use of clozapine (but note: not recommended by NICE).

Uncommon

■ Catatonia/stupor.

■ OCD.

■ Movement disorders (e.g. Parkinson's disease).

■ Neuroleptic malignant syndrome.

The last three indications were not included in the NICE remit.

Outcome/efficacy

■ ECT appears to be extremely effective in depressive disorder, with a response rate greater than that of chemical or psychological treatment at 60–80%. A recent meta-analysis confirms these findings but the trial base is of limited quality. Patients receiving ECT represent a specific population, generally more severe and 'treatment resistant' than those receiving other treatments.

■ Efficacy and cognitive side-effects appear related to the dose of current applied.

■ A direct comparison of matched patients (with random allocation) has not been made with contemporary antidepressant or psychological care.

■ Relapse rates are high (especially in treatment-resistant patients), with up to 50% of patients relapsing within the year following treatment. Additional prophylactic treatment is required and has been shown to reduce relapse.

Side-effects

■ The principal physical hazards of ECT lie with those adverse events encountered in generally following brief general anaesthesia. It is recommended that senior anaesthetists experienced in the use of ECT conduct sessions.

■ Headache and nausea are common, and respond to conventional treatment.

Cognitive impairment

■ Acute confusional state: immediately following treatment patients are typically disorientated. This lasts for about 20 minutes.

■ Anterograde amnesia: patients may experience difficulty in learning new material for a couple of months after treatment. This effect is transient, and may be of less significance than the anterograde learning difficulties seen in untreated depressive disorder.

■ Retrograde amnesia: many patients report difficulty in recalling memories that were intact prior to treatment. This is usually restricted to events just prior to each treatment, but less commonly, a significant minority of patients complain of persistent deficits extending back decades with patchy loss of autobiographical memories. This impairment is difficult to demonstrate using objective neuropsychological tests.

■ In general it is difficult to disentangle the cognitive effects of depression from those induced by ECT. Often, overall cognitive function improves as depression lifts.

■ Effects on cognitive function are cumulative throughout the course of ECT. Further treatments after symptom relief is achieved (in an effort to bolster response, for example) are not justified.

Cautions and contraindications

Absolute

■ Raised intracranial pressure.
■ Recent cerebrovascular accident.
■ Unstable vascular aneurysm.
■ Recent myocardial infarction with unstable rhythm.

Relative

■ Pregnancy.
■ Retinal detachment.
■ Cerebral tumour.
■ History of cerebrovascular accident.

References

Key references
Anderson IM, Tomenson BM. The efficacy of selective serotonin re-uptake inhibitors in depression: a meta-analysis of studies against tricyclic antidepressants. J Psychopharmacol 1994; 8:238–49

Charney DS, Menkes DB, Heninger GR. Receptor sensitivity and the mechanism of action of antidepressant treatment: implications for the etiology and therapy of depression. Arch Gen Psychiatry 1981; 38:1160

Cookson J. Side-effects of antidepressants. Br J Psychiatry 1993; 163 (Suppl. 20):20–4

Frank E, Kupfer DJ, Perel JM *et al*. Three-year outcomes for maintenance therapies in recurrent depression. Arch Gen Psychiatry 1990; 47:1093

Geddes J (for the UK ECT review group). Efficacy and safety of electroconvulsive therapy in depressive disorders: a systematic review and meta-analysis. Lancet 2003; 361:799–808

McAllister-Williams RH, Ferrier IN, Young AH. Mood and neuropsychological function in depression: the role of corticosteroids and serotonin Psychol Med 1998; 28:573–84

Meltzer HY. Serotonergic dysfunction in depression. Br J Psychiatry 1989; 155 (Suppl. 8):25

National Institute for Clinical Excellence Technology Appraisal Guidance 59. Guidance on the use of electroconvulsive therapy, 2003. http://www.nice.org.uk

Potter WZ, Rudorfer MV, Manji H. The pharmacologic treatment of depression. N Engl J Med 1991; 325:633

Preskorn SH. Pharmacokinetics of antidepressants: why and how are they relevant to treatment? J Clin Psychiatry 1993; 54 (Suppl. 9):14–34

Reid IC, Stewart CA. How antidepressants work. Br J Psychiatry 2001; 178:299–303

Stimpson N, Agrawal N, Lewis G. Randomised controlled trials investigating pharmacological and psychological interventions for treatment-refractory depression. Br J Psychiatry 2002; 181:284–94

Further reading
Anderson IM, Nutt DJ, Deakin JFW. Evidence-based guidelines for treating depressive disorders with antidepressants: a revision of the 1993 British Association for Psychopharmacology guidelines. J Psychopharmacol 2000; 14:3–20

Ashton HA. Brain Function and Psychotropic Drugs. Oxford: Oxford University Press, 1992

Freeman CP. The ECT Handbook. The second report of the Royal College of Psychiatrists' Special Committee on ECT. London: Royal College of Psychiatrists: Council Report CR39, 1995 (new report expected 2004/5)

King DJ. Seminars in Clinical Psychopharmacology. London: Gaskell, 1995 (new edition expected 2004)

5 'Mood stabilisers': lithium and anticonvulsants

What is a mood stabiliser?

■ The term 'mood stabiliser' has been applied to lithium and anticonvulsant drugs used to treat bipolar disorder. It is also starting to be applied to some atypical antipsychotics. Its use has become more controversial with developments in anticonvulsant and atypical antipsychotic use in bipolar disorder.

■ It refers to the ability of a drug to treat one or both poles of bipolar disorder without causing a switch to the other pole (cf. antidepressants which can cause a switch to mania).

■ There are however problems in its use:
  – Should it only be applied to drugs that are effective against both poles?
  – The evidence for efficacy of drugs is often clearer for one pole than the other.
  – Does it refer to acute or maintenance treatment, or both?

■ A recent suggestion is that drugs can be classified as those that treat from Above (i.e. mania), called type A mood stabilisers, those that treat from Below (i.e. depression), called type B mood stabilisers, and those that are both A and B. Some advocate simply referring to drugs' antimanic or antidepressive properties.

Lithium

History

■ Lithium is an alkaline metal element that occurs naturally as the mineral petalite. It is widely used today in swimming pool filters and batteries for mobile phones and computers.

- The Australian psychiatrist John Cade first proposed the use of lithium salts in the treatment of 'psychotic excitement' in 1949, though its sedative and depressant properties had been known since at least the preceding century.
- Lithium salts were once used extensively as a treatment for gout because lithium urate is particularly soluble and promotes the excretion of urates rather than their deposition in tissue.
- Lithium chloride was briefly used as a sodium salt substitute before its toxicity was properly appreciated.

Mechanism of action

The mode of action of lithium remains only partially understood – range of effects at a number of different levels in the central nervous system (CNS):

- Effects on cation transport.
- Effects on individual neurotransmitters.
- Effects on intracellular second messenger systems.

Effects on cation transport

- Increases the activity of Na^+/K^+ ATP-ase in patients (but, interestingly, not in healthy controls).
- May displace Ca^{2+} and Mg^{2+} ions at a range of sites relevant to neural function, e.g. modulation of Ca^{2+}-dependent activities in the CNS, such as neurotransmitter release.

Monoaminergic neurotransmission

- Increases the synthesis and release of 5-HT.
- Increases transmission at 5-HT_{1A} receptors.
- Decreases transmission at 5-HT_2 receptors.
- Enhances platelet 5-HT uptake.
- Increases NA uptake into synaptosomes.
- May reduce NA turnover overall in man.

Cholinergic neurotransmission

- Increases choline levels.
- Enhances cholinesterase inhibitor toxicity.
- Increases the growth hormone response to cholinergic agonist pyridostigmine.

These findings suggest that lithium enhances cholinergic activity in the brain. It is conceivable that these cholinomimetic effects may contribute to antimanic actions, while lithium toxicity resembles atropine poisoning.

Effects on second messengers

Lithium has many interactions with intracellular 'second messenger' systems and can thus modify signal transduction pathways:

- Inhibits Na^+-induced cAMP activity.
- Limits inositol trisphosphate (IP_3) formation.
- Reduces activity of protein kinases.

The drug can therefore alter the signal induced by multiple neurotransmitter systems, allowing mediation of complex behavioural and physiological responses (see Chapter 1). It is widely believed that these mechanisms account ultimately for the efficacy of the drug.

Neuroprotective effects

- Recent research suggests that lithium has a range of protective effects on neural function and integrity. Bipolar disorder is associated with structural brain changes and this property may play an important part in the overall efficacy of lithium.
- In animal studies and in isolated human neural cells, lithium has been shown to increase the expression of important neuroprotective proteins.
- Consistent with these effects, lithium appears to increase grey matter volume in patients with bipolar I disorder, to increase the levels of N-acetylaspartate, a putative marker of neuronal viability, in bipolar patients and healthy volunteers and to enhance neurogenesis in rat hippocampus.
- This evidence suggests that lithium may exert some of its long-term benefits in the treatment of mood disorders via neuroprotective effects and that lithium may have potential therapeutic properties in neurodegenerative disorders.

Pharmacokinetics

- Rapidly absorbed in the upper gastrointestinal tract.
- Peak serum levels being achieved within two to three hours.
- Unbound in serum.
- Excreted unchanged by the kidney at a constant rate proportional to the glomerular filtration rate.

- Steady-state is achieved after five to seven days.
- Individual lithium preparations have different bioavailability and cannot be substituted dose for dose.

Indications

Efficacy in acute mania
- In clinical trials lithium is effective in 60–80% of acutely ill patients.
- Poorer responses are seen in patients with mixed affective episodes or a rapid cycling pattern.
- Higher levels required than for prophylaxis.
- Lithium treatment for acute mania was previously considered a first-line strategy in the USA, though in Europe antipsychotic drugs have generally been used as the primary treatment in this situation. This is partly because lithium has little sedative activity of its own.
- Lithium should be used cautiously with antipsychotics because of alleged risks of neurotoxicity when lithium is combined with high doses of antipsychotic agents.

Bipolar prophylaxis
- Lithium provides effective prophylaxis against mood swings in severe and recurrent bipolar disorder in a proportion of patients. In initial randomised controlled trials, around 80% of patients were reported to benefit. More recent trials, however, suggest poorer results with 70% of patients relapsing and only 30% having good occupational outcome.
- The decision to commence prophylaxis is based on the frequency and severity of episodes. A traditional rule of thumb has been:
  - After two illnesses within two years.
  - After three illnesses in five years.
  - After one severe illness.
- Recent emphasis on the recurrent and progressive nature of bipolar disorder has increasingly led to recommending commencement of prophylaxis after a single manic episode.
- The decision to commence prophylaxis is also governed by likely compliance. Admissions for mania increased after introduction of lithium:
  - Abrupt lithium discontinuation leads to rebound mania (and thus more manic episodes than would have occurred had the drug never been started). A meta-analysis of 19 published studies on lithium discontinuation found that time to recurrence of affective disorder (mostly mania) was three months for 50% of patients.

– As a result, it has been recommended that patients must take the medication for longer than two years without discontinuation for benefits to accrue.

Efficacy in routine practice

■ Lithium is probably ineffective in approx. 40% of bipolar patients in everyday practice and there is little doubt that therapeutic use could be improved.

■ As noted above, there is an excess recurrence after withdrawal and short-term use may worsen the course of the illness.

■ Despite its long history, lithium use lacks a firm evidence base and data are particularly limited on the value of lithium in bipolar depression.

■ There is increasing evidence that lithium may help reduce suicidal ideation and prevent completed suicide.

Unipolar prophylaxis

■ Lithium is also used in the prophylaxis of recurrent unipolar depressive disorder.

■ Controlled trials suggest response rates of 30–40%, and while the strategy is significantly more efficacious than placebo, the magnitude of effect is small.

■ Continuous antidepressant prescription appears more effective than lithium prophylaxis.

Predicting response to lithium (Table 5.1)

Table 5.1 Predictors of response

Predictors of good response	Predictors of poor response
Greater adherence to treatment	Rapid cycling bipolar illness
'Pure' form of bipolar illness	Paranoid features
Endogenomorphic unipolar illness	Substance abuse
Family history of bipolar illness	Poor psychosocial support
Mania followed by depression	Depression followed by mania
Previous good response to treatment	

Using lithium

Initiating therapy

Prior to commencing lithium therapy:

■ It is important to establish the degree of affective morbidity, both to clarify the indication for therapy and as a reference baseline against which outcome may be judged.

■ Because of the danger of rebound mania following discontinuation, the need for prolonged treatment (at least two years) should be discussed.

Relevant investigations include:

■ Renal function (serum creatinine; full creatinine clearance usually only needed if there are concerns about renal function).

■ Thyroid function.

■ ECG (especially if there are cardiac concerns).

■ Weight.

■ Pregnancy test for females in the years of reproductive potential.

Dosing

■ A sensible starting dose is 600–800 mg at night for otherwise healthy individuals.

■ Try to use single daily dosing – divided dosing complicates serum level assessment and may increase the risk of renal toxicity.

■ The serum lithium concentration level should be determined after five to seven days, and the dose adjusted to achieve a value between 0.5–1.0 mmol/l.

■ Concentrations between 0.8 and 1.0 mmol/l are usually needed for the acute treatment of mania. For prophylaxis some patients may achieve good therapeutic results with concentrations as low as 0.4 mmol/l.

Monitoring treatment

■ Mood should be monitored conscientiously (a mood diary may be helpful).

■ Ask about adherence at each assessment.

■ Weight.

■ A reasonable schedule for blood monitoring is:
  – serum lithium level every three months;
  – renal function every six months;
  – thyroid function every six months to one year.

- ECG if cardiac concerns.
- If it becomes necessary to discontinue lithium this should be done slowly in an effort to reduce the likelihood of rebound episodes of illness.

Use in pregnancy and lactation
- Reported to induce teratogenic defects in <11% of births, most commonly Ebstein's anomaly.
- If lithium use is necessary during pregnancy, close monitoring is advised, as is liaison with the obstetrician.
- Lithium should be stopped at the onset of labour and reintroduced in the first week post-partum
- Lithium is excreted into breast milk and so breast-feeding is not advised.

Adverse effects of lithium

Many of the adverse effects are related to serum concentration and may be minimised if levels are kept below 0.8 mmol/l.

Side-effects
- Thirst, polydipsia, polyuria.
- Gastrointestinal problems – nausea, diarrhoea.
- Weight gain.
- Tremor.
- Precipitates or worsens skin problems.
- Mild impairment of attention and memory.
- T-wave flattening/inversion in 30% of patients.
- Hypothyroidism and nontoxic goitre (5%).
- Impaired renal function (see below):
  - impaired renal tubular function (5–10%);
  - impaired glomerular function (possible).
- Leucocytosis.

Effects on renal function
- Inhibits the action of antidiuretic hormone on the kidney and reduces the ability to concentrate urine causing polyuria (and consequent thirst/poly-dipsia):
  - Paradoxically, may be improved by treatment with the diuretic amiloride.
- The long-term effects of lithium on renal function are controversial:
  - Polyuria does not predict lasting renal damage.
  - Although an early, uncontrolled study found that 21% of patients who

had been treated with lithium for more than 15 years had a reduced glomerular filtration rate, subsequent controlled studies demonstrated few differences between treated and untreated patients with respect to renal pathology.

Lithium toxicity

Lithium has a low and narrow therapeutic index, hence the need for regular monitoring. Signs of toxicity appear generally at levels above 1.3 mmol/l though they can occur within the 'therapeutic range' in some individuals.

- Early features include:
  - An exacerbation of existing side-effects.
  - Nausea, vomiting, diarrhoea.
  - Tremor.
- As toxicity develops further:
  - Disorientation.
  - Dysarthria.
  - Convulsions.
  - Coma.
  - Death from cardiac effects or pulmonary complications.
- Treatment of lithium toxicity:
  - Lithium toxicity represent a potentially serious and life-threatening medical emergency.
  - Admission may be required, for rehydration and the administration of anticonvulsants, depending on severity.
  - Haemodialysis may be necessary where serum levels exceed 3.0 mm/l, coma supervenes, or there is no response to supportive measures over 24 hours.

Drug interactions with lithium

Table 5.2 Drug interactions

Increased lithium levels	CNS toxicity
Diuretics	Antidepressants
Nonsteroidal anti-inflammatory drugs (NSAIDs)	Antipsychotics
Angiotensin-converting enzyme (ACE) inhibitors	Antihypertensives
	General anaesthetics?

Mortality of treated patients

- Bipolar illness carries an excess mortality.
- Lithium treatment reduces the standardised mortality rate to a level similar to the general population.
- Estimated to increase life expectancy by about seven years.
- Increased mortality rate returns after stopping treatment.

Other indications

- Adjunct to antidepressants in depression.
- Prevention of puerperal psychosis.
- Prophylaxis in schizoaffective disorder and cyclical schizophrenia.
- Adjunct to antipsychotics in schizophrenia.
- Reduction in impulsivity.
- Reversal of neutropenia.

Anticonvulsants

Background

- The use of anticonvulsants is increasing in affective disorder. However, the mood-stabilising properties of anticonvulsants may not be mediated by the same mechanisms that mediate seizure control in epilepsy.
- The use of anticonvulsants in bipolar disorder has led to speculation about the possibility of a common pathophysiology between epilepsy and severe psychotic disorder. Processes that appear to be similar to kindling phenomena occur in the natural history of bipolar and unipolar affective disorders. Most anticonvulsant drugs with mood-stabilising properties also inhibit the electrically induced kindling of seizure activity in animals.
- The precise pharmacological properties which account for their efficacy is uncertain. In general such drugs enhance the actions of GABA and thus strengthen inhibitory circuits in the CNS. It is possible that their therapeutic actions are mediated through effects on membrane excitability.
- The antisuicidal effects seen with lithium do not appear to apply to anticonvulsants.
- ECT therapy, which is also a potent anticonvulsant, has powerful antidepressive and antimanic actions.

Sodium valproate

■ Available in different formulations. Valproate semisodium (divalproex sodium in the USA) is a mixture of sodium valproate and valproic acid and is now licensed in the UK for the treatment of acute mania.

■ It is the most frequently prescribed 'mood stabiliser' in the USA.

■ Increasingly used in Europe.

■ No longer restricted to patients who have failed to respond to or are intolerant of lithium, but is increasingly being used as first-line monotherapy.

Mode of action

■ Enhances GABAergic function.

■ Inhibits GABA-transaminase.

■ Increases GABA binding in some brain structures, most notably the hippocampus.

■ Like lithium, inhibits the formation of protein kinase C.

■ Reduces the action of NA at $\alpha_2$adrenoceptors.

■ May antagonise the functional effects of DA.

Indications

■ Increasing use as a first-line antimanic agent.

■ Treatment-refractory mania.

■ Rapid cycling bipolar disorder.

■ Most effective in nonpsychotic patients.

■ Although promising, further data are required before definitive statements can be made about the value of valproate in prophylaxis.

■ In epilepsy, valproate is used to treat primary generalised seizures, generalised absences and myoclonic seizures.

Adverse effects

■ Nausea and vomiting.

■ Blood dyscrasias.

■ Hepatotoxicity.

■ Tremor.

■ Weight gain.

■ Alopecia.

■ ?Polycystic ovaries and infertility in women.

■ Teratogenicity:
  – heart;
  – neural tube;
  – lip and palate.

Valproate use in practice

■ The monitoring of clinical conditions, especially mood and weight are important.

■ It is unclear if serum concentrations are a useful guide to dose but may be helpful in cases of poor response/compliance.

■ Valproate semisodium and other valproate preparations do not have the same dose equivalence (higher bioavailability with valproate semisodium).

■ Monitoring of liver and clotting function (including platelets) is required if there are clinical concerns or surgery.

■ Folate supplementation should be considered in women of childbearing age.

Carbamazepine

Mode of action

The therapeutic effect of carbamazepine may be mediated via the adenylate cyclase and phosphoinositol second-messenger systems.

Indications

■ The evidence base for the efficacy of carbamazepine in treating mania, bipolar depression and in prophylaxis is extremely limited. In recent studies it appears less effective than lithium.

■ Limited evidence suggests that carbamazepine may be effective in treatment-resistant mania and treatment-resistant schizophrenia.

■ It is used as an adjunct to lithium in the prophylaxis of bipolar affective disorder and has been considered to have particular value in rapid-cycling bipolar disorder.

■ Although the drug enjoys a reputation for efficacy in recurrent unipolar illness and treatment-resistant depressive disorder, there is little convincing evidence to support this.

Adverse effects

Although widely regarded by British psychiatrists as a 'safer' alternative to lithium, carbamazepine has a range of potentially serious side-effects and patient tolerance is poor (Table 5.3). Many of the autoimmune effects are thought to be related to the metabolite carbamazepine-10,11-epoxide.

Table 5.3 *Adverse effects of carbamazepine*

CNS	Headache, dizziness, drowsiness, diplopia
Liver	Elevation of hepatic enzymes, hepatitis, cholestatic jaundice
Gastrointestinal	Nausea, vomiting
Blood dyscrasias	
Skin rashes	
Teratogenic effects	(?Secondary to folate deficiency)

Interactions

Carbamazepine has important pharmacokinetic interactions.

■ It induces the metabolism of:
  - anticoagulants;
  - antidepressants;
  - antipsychotics;
  - oral contraceptives (leading to contraceptive failure);
  - steroids.

■ Other interactions occur with alcohol, analgesics, antibacterials, Ca^{2+} channel blockers and ulcer-healing drugs.

Oxcarbazepine

■ Related to carbamazepine and has a common active metabolite, 10,11-dihydroxycarbamazepine.

■ Compared with carbamazepine:
  - It is not metabolised to carbamazepine-10,11-epoxide and lacks the same propensity to cause autoimmune reactions and rashes.
  - It causes less hepatic enzyme induction.

■ There is a small controlled trial suggesting antimanic efficacy but only limited open-study evidence in prophylaxis and its place in the treatment of bipolar disorder is unclear.

Lamotrigine

■ Effective as augmentation therapy for patients with refractory epilepsy.

■ It has a novel mechanism of action, stabilising neuronal membranes and reducing the release of excitatory amino acids (particularly glutamate) by blocking voltage-dependent Na^+ channels.

■ Lamotrigine has been shown to be antidepressant in bipolar depression as monotherapy.

■ Lamotrigine has shown efficacy in rapid cycling bipolar disorder and prevents relapse into bipolar depression after index episodes of both mania and bipolar depression where it may be more effective than lithium.

■ It appears to lack antimanic efficacy.

■ It can cause severe rash and Stevens–Johnson syndrome. The risk is reduced by very slow dose titration.

■ Its metabolism is inhibited by sodium valproate so even slower dose titration and lower final doses are required in patients on valproate.

Other anticonvulsants

Topiramate

■ A new anticonvulsant drug that is used as adjunctive therapy for partial onset seizures.

■ It enhances GABA activity and blocks glutamate at non-NMDA receptors.

■ It has not shown antimanic efficacy in controlled trials.

■ Preliminary open observations of adjunctive topiramate treatment suggest that it may have antimanic or anticycling effects in some patients with bipolar disorder including those who are treatment resistant.

■ It causes appetite suppression and weight loss.

Gabapentin

■ In use as augmentation therapy in patients with partial seizures resistant to conventional therapies.

■ Structurally related to GABA with an unknown mechanism of action.

■ Gabapentin has been of particular interest because it possesses a wide therapeutic index and a relatively benign side-effect profile. Side-effects reported with gabapentin are transient and minor, the most common being somnolence, dizziness, ataxia and fatigue. It is not associated with hepatic or haematological problems.

■ The use of gabapentin in rapid cycling bipolar disorder, mania and bipolar depression has been suggested by open trials, but these findings have not been replicated in two randomised controlled trials.

■ It is effective against anxiety symptoms in bipolar disorder.

Tiagabine

■ A novel anticonvulsant which reduces the re-uptake of GABA into neuronal and glial cells.

■ Elevated brain levels of GABA have been reported in patients with euthymic bipolar disorder using nuclear magnetic spectroscopy and therefore in theory this may be reversed by tiagabine.

■ Preliminary case reports have yielded conflicting results.

Levetiracetam
■ Novel anticonvulsant used as adjunctive therapy for partial-onset seizures with unknown mechanism of action.
■ There is equivocal open evidence in mania.

Zonisamide
■ Novel anticonvulsant used as adjunctive therapy for partial-onset seizures.
■ Blocks Na^+ and Ca^{2+} channels and is a weak carbonic anhydrase inhibitor. It facilitiates DA and 5-HT function.
■ Currently under investigation in bipolar disorder.
■ It causes weight loss when used in adjunctive therapy.

Antipsychotics

See Chapter 3.
■ Typical and atypical antipsychotics are widely used in bipolar disorder.
■ Antipsychotics are effective antimanic agents. Traditionally they have been first-line agents in acute mania in Europe whereas lithium, anticonvulsants and benzodiazepines have been preferred in the USA.
■ Side-effects associated with older typical antipsychotics, and concern that they may cause depression, have meant that their use has been discouraged in prophylaxis.
■ Recent evidence with atypical antipsychotics (particularly olanzapine) has confirmed acute antimanic effects, suggested possible antidepressant properties and shown efficacy in prophylaxis. Olanzapine has now been licensed in the UK for the prophylaxis of bipolar disorder. The term 'mood stabiliser' is increasingly being applied to atypical antipsychotics used in this way.

Antidepressants

See Chapter 4.
■ The use of antidepressants has been discouraged because of their ability to switch patients into mania, hence they are not viewed as mood stabilisers.
■ Switch rates appear highest with TCAs, MAOIs and possibly dual-action re-uptake inhibitors such as venlafaxine and lowest with SSRIs, which are the preferred group if an antidepressant is indicated.
■ Antidepressants should not be used in bipolar disorder without concomitant use of an antimanic agent.

■ The role of antidepressants is being re-evaluated and the long-term use of antidepressants in some bipolar patients may be beneficial.

Benzodiazepines (BDZs)

See Chapter 6.

Although BDZs are useful in adjunctive treatment of manic excitement and agitation there is no evidence they treat the underlying mood disorder.

Treatment issues

■ The treatment of bipolar disorder is relatively under-researched in relation to schizophrenia and depression, in particular the treatment of bipolar II disorder and bipolar spectrum disorders.

■ Treatment is complicated by the often chaotic nature of the illness with different phases and presentations.

■ Continuing symptoms and impaired functioning are common between major relapses.

■ Only a minority of patients can be maintained on a single agent such as lithium but at present there is limited evidence about the most effective way to combine different agents.

■ In the UK the National Institute for Clinical Excellence (NICE) has given guidance supporting the use of olanzapine and valproate semisodium in acute mania. NICE guidelines on the treatment of bipolar disorder are expected in June 2006.

References

Key references
Bauer M, Dopfmer S. Lithium augmentation in treatment-resistant depression: meta-analysis of placebo-controlled studies. J Clin Psychopharmacol 1999; 19:427–34
Coryell W, Winokur G, Solomon D *et al*. Lithium and recurrence in a long-term follow-up of bipolar affective disorder. Psychol Med 1997; 27:281–9.
Goodwin GM for the Consensus Group of the British Association for Psychopharmacology. Evidence-based guidelines for treating bipolar disorder: recommendations from the British Association for Psychopharmacology. J Psychopharmacol 2003; 17:149–73
Lenox RH, McNamara RK, Papke RL, Manji HK. Neurobiology of lithium: an update. J Clin Psychiatry 2000; 61:5–15
Manji H, Lenox R. Signaling: cellular insights into the pathophysiology of bipolar disorder. Biol Psychiatry 2000; 48:518–30
Thase M, Sachs G. Bipolar depression: pharmacotherapy and related therapeutic strategies. Biol Psychiatry 2000; 48:558–72

Tondo L, Hennen J, Baldessarini RJ. Lower suicide risk with long-term lithium treatment in major affective illness: a meta-analysis. Acta Psychiatr Scand 2001; 104:163–72

Young AH, Macritchie KA, Calabrese JR. Treatment of bipolar affective disorder. New drug treatments are emerging, but more clinical evidence is required. BMJ 2000; 321(7272):1302–3

Further reading

Dichter MA, Brodie MJ. New antiepileptic drugs. N Engl J Med 1996; 334(24):1583–90

Drevets W, Gadde K, Krishnan K. Neuroimaging studies of mood disorders. In: Neurobiology of Mental Illness (Charney D, Nestler E, Bunney B, eds) Oxford: Oxford University Press, 1999; pp 394–418

Goodwin F, Ghaemi S. The impact of the discovery of lithium on psychiatric thought and practice in the USA and Europe. Aust NZ J Psychiatry 1999; 33:S54–S64

National Institute for Clinical Excellence Technology Appraisal Guidance 66. Olanzapine and valproate semisodium in the treatment of acute mania associated with bipolar I disorder, 2003. http://www.nice.org.uk

Post R. Mood disorders: Treatment of bipolar disorders. In: Kaplan & Sadock's Comprehensive Textbook of Psychiatry (Sadock B, Sadock V, eds) New York: Williams & Wilkins, 2000; pp 1385–430

6 Anxiolytics

History

■ *Pre-benzodiazepine era:* bromides, chloral and paraldehyde introduced in the 19th century and barbiturates, meprobamate in the 20th century but problems with low therapeutic index. Barbiturates predominated until introduction of benzodiazepines (BDZs).

■ *Benzodiazepine era:* chlordiazepoxide (1960) followed by diazepam with rapid growth in use, peaking about 1979. Higher therapeutic index than barbiturates but addiction and withdrawal problems at usual therapeutic doses fully recognised in 1981, leading to reduced prescribing (Table 6.1):

– in 1978, 10% of men and 20% of women given a BDZ; 15% for >4 weeks, 1.5% for >1 year. *Anxiety*: peak prescribing 50–65 years, *hypnotics*: peak prescribing 65+ years. Long-term use associated with elderly, multiple, chronic physical disorders;

– hypnotic prescriptions have remained fairly constant at 10–12 million per annum.

■ *Post-benzodiazepine era*: alternatives to benzodiazepines developed that are less/non-addictive, e.g. serotonergic drugs, BDZ partial agonists, GABA/ peptidergic drugs, but BDZs remain frequently used.

Table 6.1 Benzodiazepine prescribing in the UK

Year	UK scripts for hypnotics and tranquillisers	Comments
1960	27 million	15 million barbiturates
1974	40 million	25 million benzodiazepines
1979	31 million	Few for barbiturates
1990	16 million	12 million hypnotics

Neurobiology

Brain aversion system

- Periaqueductal grey (PAG):
  - brainstem area;
  - linked to stereotyped, 'hard-wired' responses of fight or flight;
  - panic attacks likely to be linked to activation of PAG – spontaneous panics may originate at this level.
- Medial hypothalamus:
  - autonomic and endocrine components of anxiety response.
- Amygdala:
  - important role in classical conditioning and co-ordinating/integrating fear responses;
  - response to cues and close threat (e.g. startle reactions) with inputs from thalamus;
  - likely to be involved in phobias and post-traumatic stress disorder (PTSD).
- Septohippocampal system:
  - role in context of anxiety and inhibition of behaviour;
  - likely role in avoidance and anticipatory anxiety.
- Temporal and prefrontal cortex:
  - higher order processing, including of social situations;
  - likely role in anticipatory and socially induced anxiety.

Neurochemical theories

Noradrenaline (NA)

- Stimulation of the major brain NA nucleus, the locus coeruleus (LC) in animals gives an anxiety-like state.
- Physiological symptoms of anxiety in man are consistent with adrenergic overactivity.
- Yohimbine (α_2 antagonist) infusion increases NA release and causes panic in panic disorder patients but has little effect in non-anxious subjects.
- Clonidine (α_2 agonist) infusion causes decreased NA release and may decrease anxiety in some situations.
- β-Adrenoceptor antagonists reduce physiological symptoms of anxiety.

Serotonin (5-HT)

- 5-HT$_{1A}$ partial agonists (e.g. buspirone) can decrease anxiety in generalised anxiety disorder (GAD) but are not effective in panic disorder.
- Some 5-HT$_2$ agonists (e.g. *m*-chlorophenylpiperazine) are anxiogenic.
- SSRIs are effective in treating a wide range of anxiety disorders – GAD, panic disorder, social anxiety disorder, PTSD, obsessive–compulsive disorder (OCD) – but can make anxiety symptoms worse in the initial phase of treatment of panic disorder.
- Animal models of anxiety show complex role for 5-HT system.
- Human studies suggest 5-HT stimulation reduces panic anxiety but increases generalised anxiety.
- 5-HT acts at different levels of the brain aversion system, inhibiting brainstem hard-wired panic system but increasing anxiety in temporal lobe structures involved in condition/generalised anxiety.
- In addition there is 'crosstalk' between neurotransmitters, e.g. one theory: ↑5-HT release → ↑frontal cortex stimulation → ↓ activity of GABA projection to LC → ↑LC firing.

GABA

- BDZs (which enhance GABA function) effective in treatment of anxiety.
- Pentylenetetrazol (inhibitor of GABA$_A$–BDZ receptor) causes extreme anxiety symptoms and seizures.
- Flumazenil (BDZ inhibitor) may cause panic in panic patients but not in non-anxious subjects (possibly indicates an abnormality of BDZ receptor sensitivity in panic disorder).
- BDZ receptor numbers (measured by PET studies of flumazenil binding) reduced by 20% in panic disorder patients.
- Mice genetically altered to have only 50% of γ_2 subunits (linked to BDZ binding site) in GABA$_A$–BDZ receptors (receptor 'knockout') have behavioural equivalent of anxiety.
- Effect of BDZs may involve acting on receptors on monoamine neurones, e.g. brainstem and LC leading to reduced NA and 5-HT neuronal firing.

Carbon dioxide (CO$_2$)

- Increased sensitivity to inhaled CO$_2$ in panic disorder leading to panic anxiety (but paradoxically voluntary hyperventilation, causing hypocapnia, can also induce panic).
- Lactate infusion (possibly by altering acid–base balance) provokes panic in anxious patients but not in controls.

■ The finding is consistent with possible alteration of brainstem sensitivity to CO_2.

Cholecystokinin (CCK)

■ Infusion of CCK_4 (an agonist at CCK_B receptors) induces panic.
■ CCK_B receptor antagonists anxiolytic in some animal models.

Drug treatment of anxiety

In the UK, National Institute for Clinical Excellence (NICE) guidelines for treating panic disorder and GAD are due to be published in late 2004.

Benzodiazepines

BDZs act at the $GABA_A$–BDZ receptor complex (see Chapter 1 and Fig. 6.1).
■ Endogenous ligands identified but their functional status is unknown.
■ The $GABA_A$–BDZ complex consists of five subunits from seven families of subunits (α, β, γ, δ, ϵ, π, ρ) each of which contains a number of subtypes of units. The most common type of $GABA_A$–BDZ receptor (50% of total) contains two α_1, two β_2 and one γ_2 subunit (see Fig. 6.1) arranged around the Cl^- ion channel.
■ GABA is the main inhibitory transmitter in the CNS. Two GABA molecules are required to increase Cl^- ion channel conductance (by increasing the time the channel is open). This reduces the likelihood of an action potential.
■ The BDZ binding site is at the junction between α_1 and γ_2 subunits (see Fig. 6.1).
■ When a BDZ occupies its own receptor it enhances the action of GABA at its receptor resulting in greater flow of Cl^- into the neurone.
■ If GABA is absent or the receptor is blocked, e.g. by bicuculline, then BDZs on their own will have no effect, making them relatively safe in overdose (cf. barbiturates, which can open the channel in the absence of GABA resulting in respiratory depression).
■ Type I BDZ receptors are mainly found in the cerebellum and are related to induction and maintenance of sleep whereas type II BDZ receptors tend to be found in the spinal cord and limbic regions and are associated with muscle relaxant, anxiolytic and anticonvulsant effects.
■ Newer hypnotic drugs modulate the $GABA_A$–BDZ receptor complex but have pharmacodynamic differences to BDZ:

– zolpidem (an imadazopyridine) and zaleplon (a pyrazolopyrimidine) are relatively selective for the type I receptor;
– zopiclone (a cyclopyrrolone) binds to a different site on the $GABA_A$–BDZ receptor complex from standard BDZs and zolpidem.

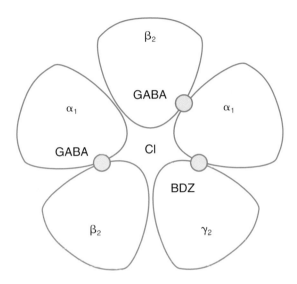

Figure 6.1 *$GABA_A$–benzodiazepine receptor complex showing subunits and binding sites of ligands (binding sites for GABA and BDZ shown ◯).*

Agonist/inverse agonist effects (Table 6.2)

Table 6.2 *Range of effects possible for drugs active at the BDZ receptor*

Full agonist	Partial agonist	Neutral antagonist	Partial inverse agonist	Full inverse agonist
Action				
Sedative	Mild sedation	No effect		
Anxiolytic	Mild anxiolytic	of	Anxiogenic	Anxiogenic
Anticonvulsant	Anticonvulsant	its own		Pro-convulsant
Example				
Diazepam	Clonazepam	Flumazenil	(Flumazenil in patients with panic disorder)	Ethyl-β-carboline-3-carboxylate (β-CCE) FG7142

■ BDZ effects are through modulation of GABA function. The BDZs are unusual in having inhibitory and stimulatory effects on GABA function.

■ Full agonists (e.g. diazepam) and partial agonists at the BDZ receptor act to *enhance* the action of GABA.

■ Full and partial inverse agonists *inhibit* the action of GABA. They act in the opposite way to a typical BDZ and reduce Cl⁻ influx. There are no clinically useful drugs in this category at present. However, in patients with panic disorder, flumazenil may act like a partial inverse agonist and cause an increase in anxiety symptoms.

■ Neutral antagonists occupy BDZ receptor and prevent agonists or inverse agonists interacting with it. Flumazenil does this under most circumstances.

Effects of benzodiazepines (Table 6.3)

Table 6.3 *Principal actions of benzodiazepines*

Action	Use
Anxiolytic	Anxiety disorders, alcohol withdrawal, premedication in anaesthesia
Hypnotic	Sleep disorder
Anticonvulsant	Epilepsy, myoclonus, alcohol withdrawal
Muscle relaxant	Muscle spasticity, akathisia
Amnesic	Premedication
Impair psychomotor function	

■ Little direct effect on autonomic, cardiovascular or respiratory function unless given intravenously.

■ No hepatic enzyme induction.

Clinical efficacy of benzodiazepines in psychiatric disorders

■ Sleep:
  – pharmacokinetic properties important (see below); shorter elimination half-life compounds preferred;
  – newer compounds with different pharmacodynamics to classical BDZs (zolpidem, zopiclone, zaleplon) are claimed to cause less dependence/withdrawal;
  – very short half-life compounds (zaleplon) are only useful for sleep induction and not sleep maintenance;

- in the UK the National Institute for Clinical Excellence (NICE) has recently (2004) given guidance that there is no compelling evidence to distinguish between the newer compounds and shorter-acting BDZ hypnotics. This is disputed by some user groups and experts due to longer half-lives of BDZ hypnotics (see Table 6.6).

■ Anxiety disorders:
  - longer half-life drugs indicated; short half-life more prone to withdrawal problems;
  - BDZs effective in 'core' anxiety disorders; efficacy seems to be maintained for many patients with GAD and panic disorder; some may develop tolerance;
  - not believed to be effective as primary treatment for longer-term treatment of other anxiety disorders such as social phobia, specific phobias, OCD, PTSD but few long-term clinical trials.

■ Alcohol withdrawal and epilepsy:
  - longer half-life drugs indicated.

Adverse effects of benzodiazepines (Table 6.4)

Table 6.4 Main adverse effects. The context of use determines whether these are wanted or unwanted

Frequency	Adverse effect
Common	Drowsiness, dizziness, psychomotor impairment
Occasional	Dry mouth, blurred vision, gastrointestinal upset, headache, increased risk of falls in the elderly
Rare	Amnesia, restlessness, disinhibition, skin rash, eosinophilia

Pharmacokinetics (Table 6.5)

Table 6.5 Main pharmacokinetic properties, using diazepam as the example

Parameter	Findings for diazepam
Bioavailability	Almost complete with oral dose
Peak concentration	30–90 minutes after single dose
Protein binding	95%
Renal excretion	Negligible for unchanged drug
Metabolism	Phase I to active metabolite Phase II for inactivation
Elimination half-life	Young adults: 20 h Elderly: 30–100 h Phase I metabolite: desmethyldiazepam: 30–90 h

■ Many BDZs undergo Phase I metabolism to produce active metabolites which:
- generally have a much longer elimination half-life than the parent compound;
- lead to prolonged effects as their plasma concentration gradually rises;
- are often largely responsible for 'hangover' effects when using BDZ regularly as a hypnotic;
- may contribute to confusion in susceptible subjects (e.g. the elderly).

■ Compounds lacking Phase I metabolism with short elimination half-lives are preferred as hypnotics (but note nitrazepam in Table 6.6 which has historically been used as a hypnotic).

Table 6.6 *Pharmacokinetic parameters for a number of BDZs and similar compounds*

Drug	Absorption	Half-life (parent drug) (h)	Metabolic phases	Half-life (active metabolite) (h)	Clinical use
Diazepam	Rapid	20–100	I+II	30–90	Anxiolytic
Alprazolam	Intermediate	5–15	I+II	Very low concentration	Antipanic
Lorazepam	Intermediate	10–20	II only	None	Anxiolytic
Nitrazepam	Intermediate	24	I+II	30–90	Hypnotic
Flurazepam	Rapid	2	I+II	30–100	Hypnotic
Temazepam	Slow	10	II only	None	Hypnotic
Zolpidem	Rapid	2	II only	None	Hypnotic
Zopiclone	Rapid	4	I+II	3–6	Hypnotic
Zaleplon	Rapid	1	II only	None	Hypnotic

Tolerance (see also Chapter 2)

■ Increased rapid eye movement sleep amount and intensity (*REM rebound*) is one example of the development of tolerance to the effects of BDZ when used as a hypnotic:
- BDZs reduce REM sleep from 25% to 10–15% of total sleep time at night with tolerance occurring within about two weeks (REM% returns to normal);
- sudden discontinuation of BDZ leads to a rebound increase in REM sleep resulting in periods of waking through the night (can take up to six weeks to return to normal);
- this leads to the patient believing they require to continue the hypnotic drug and the development of physical dependence.

■ Tolerance to different effects of BDZs not entirely clear – evidence suggests the following:
  – *Animals*: tolerance occurs to sedation, ataxia, muscle relaxation, anti-convulsant effects but less clear for 'anxiolytic' effects.
  – *Humans:* tolerance to sedation, anticonvulsant and EEG effects but less clear for psychomotor, anxiolytic and hypnotic effects.
■ Cross-tolerance may occur to other BDZs and alcohol.
■ The mechanism of tolerance with BDZs are not entirely clear but likely to be a combination of pharmacodynamic and cognitive/behavioural factors.

Benzodiazepine withdrawal syndrome (Table 6.7)
■ First fully described by Petursson and Lader (1981).
■ Previously recognised following prolonged, high-dose treatment but they described it following shorter periods of standard doses.
■ Probably affects 45% on cessation or dose reduction.
■ Personality variables have some predictive value: more common in a dependent personality.

Table 6.7 Symptoms of benzodiazepine withdrawal

Anxiety-type symptoms	Disturbance of perception	Severe but rare symptoms
Anxiety	Hypersensitivity to stimuli	Paranoid psychosis
Dysphoria	Abnormal bodily sensation	Depressive episode
Tremor	Sense of body sway	Seizures
Muscle pains	Depersonalisation	
Sleep disturbance	Visual disturbances	
Headache		
Nausea, anorexia		
Sweating		
Fatigue		

Management of benzodiazepine withdrawal syndrome:

■ gradually decrease BDZ dose over 4 to 16 weeks;
■ transfer to longer half-life drug, e.g. diazepam;
■ β-blockers can reduce severity of symptoms but do not appear to improve outcome;
■ monitor for increased alcohol consumption;
■ outcome:
  – most succeed initially;

  – one-third have some relapse but later succeed;
  – one-third fully relapse and remain on BDZs.

Toxicity in overdose
■ Patients have survived overdoses of >2 g. Psychomotor impairment has been detected for some weeks afterwards.
■ Treatment:
  – supportive therapy and gastric lavage if appropriate;
  – dialysis is probably of limited value given the large volume of distribution of these drugs;
  – flumazenil will counteract sedation but beware of its short half-life.

Benzodiazepines in pregnancy
■ Reports of cleft lip and cleft palate in uncontrolled studies.
■ Respiratory depression in the newborn of mothers on BDZs. Developmental dysmorphism (e.g. fetal alcohol syndrome) reported in 1987. However, study complicated by mothers' alcohol use. Findings not replicated in a 1992 study.

Place in clinical practice and prescribing guidelines
■ BDZs are most effective for acute anxiety states and GAD.
■ Where possible, identify causes of anxiety or insomnia and treat these appropriately.
■ Reserve BDZs for more severe symptoms.
■ Use the lowest effective dose.
■ Ideally only prescribe for two weeks and at most four weeks. Caution needed if considered for chronic anxiety where prescription may be required for more than two to four weeks.
■ Avoid 'repeat' prescriptions as far as possible.
■ Warn patients about the possibility of dependence.

5-HT$_{1A}$ receptor agonists
Background
■ Buspirone available (5-HT$_{1A}$ receptor partial agonist). Others in development (ipsapirone, gepirone) have not come to market.
■ Buspirone causes a complex cascade of events in 5-HT system: initially effect at somatodendritic receptor causes decrease in 5-HT release but effects mitigated by postsynaptic receptor agonism; chronic treatment (>2

weeks) results in return to normal of 5-HT neuronal firing and release. Combined with direct postsynaptic effect may lead to overall increase in 5-HT activity.

■ Elimination half-life is short (three hours) so requires multiple daily dosing. Slow-release form has effective half-life of nine hours. Active metabolite 1-pyramidyl piperazine (1-PP, an α_2 antagonist) may contribute to buspirone's effect.

Efficacy
■ Trials demonstrate effectiveness for GAD but not panic disorder.
■ No consistent evidence for other anxiety disorders.
■ Some evidence for better effect if patients *not* previously exposed to BDZs.
■ Also evidence for effectiveness for depression.

Adverse effects
■ Nausea, dizziness, headache.
■ No evidence of a withdrawal syndrome.
■ No interaction with alcohol.

Place in clinical practice
■ Used for GAD especially if associated symptoms of depression.
■ Does not appear to be as effective as BDZs and take longer to act. Thus of little use for acute anxiety.

Antidepressants
Background
■ TCAs were used for many years in the management of anxiety, though no large-sized randomised controlled trials (RCTs) until the 1980s.
■ MAOIs used for so-called 'atypical depression', which has had different definitions but historically includes mild/moderate depressive states with a large anxiety component (however DSM-IV definition does not specify anxiety; see Chapter 4).
■ Clomipramine demonstrated to be of benefit for OCD.
■ Clomipramine and imipramine demonstrated to benefit panic disorder.
■ More recently there have been extensive trials with the SSRIs in GAD, panic disorder and social phobia.
■ Venlafaxine, a dual NA and 5-HT re-uptake inhibitor, is active in GAD.

Mode of action and adverse effects

- See Chapter 4 for details of pharmacodynamic effects of antidepressants and their adverse effects.
- Efficacy in anxiety disorders probably related to their effects on the 5-HT system.

Efficacy

- RCTs have demonstrated efficacy of TCAs for anxiety associated with depression, GAD, panic disorder (clomipramine, imipramine) and OCD (clomipramine only).
- Clinical trials with SSRIs show efficacy across the range of anxiety disorders.

Place in clinical practice

- SSRIs first line for GAD, PTSD, social phobia, panic disorder and OCD.
- Serotonergic TCAs second line for panic disorder (clomipramine, imipramine) and OCD (clomipramine).
- In the first two weeks of treatment with an SSRI panic symptoms may worsen and may be treated with short-term BDZ.

β-Adrenoceptor antagonists

Background

- Series of classical trials in the 1960s demonstrated that there was an effect on anxiety symptoms that was due to a peripheral effect (practolol) on β-adrenoceptors (use of D and L isomers).
- Anxiety associated with thyrotoxicosis shown to respond.
- Not clear if effect is mainly through β_1 or β_2 adrenoceptors.

Efficacy

- Ten small studies, some placebo controlled, consistently show benefit for situational/performance anxiety.
- Studies to date suggest only limited efficacy in GAD.
- Ineffective in panic disorder from limited evidence.
- Attenuate severity of BDZ withdrawal symptoms.

Adverse effects

- May get hypotension from bradycardia.
- Excessive dreaming.
- Can aggravate bronchospasm, cardiac failure.
- Some observational evidence of depression of mood but not consistent.

Place in clinical practice

■ First line for situational/performance anxiety.

■ May help some GAD/panic disorder patients with many physiological symptoms of anxiety.

■ Also of value for akathisia and lithium-induced fine tremor (*not* toxicity).

Low-dose antipsychotics

■ These have been used from the 1950s, mainly thioridazine (but licence now limited to schizophrenia requiring ECG monitoring) and chlorpromazine.

■ Very few clinical trials and most are small and not placebo controlled. Weak evidence of equal efficacy to BDZ in GAD.

■ Risk of extrapyramidal side-effects and, with long-term use, tardive dyskinesia.

■ Useful for short-term use in the treatment of anxiety/agitation in association with severe depressive disorder.

■ Place of atypical antipsychotics not established.

■ Should only be considered as a last resort for some GAD patients.

Other/new approaches

■ 5-HT$_2$ antagonists appear to have efficacy in GAD but not panic disorder (which then may exacerbate). No 5-HT$_2$ antagonists are marketed for anxiety disorders but antidepressants with 5-HT$_2$ antagonism include trazodone, mirtazapine and nefazodone.

■ CCK antagonists have not shown evidence for efficacy in clinical trials. Bioavailability is a problem with these compounds.

■ CRF can be anxiogenic and CRF$_1$ antagonists may be anxiolytic. Bioavailability is a problem with these compounds.

■ Neurokinin (NK, substance P) can be anxiogenic in laboratory animals. NK$_1$ antagonists are anxiolytic in some animal models where they are not as potent as BDZs but better than SSRIs.

■ Pregabalin, which acts on a subunit of the voltage-gated Ca^{2+} channel, shows some evidence of effect in clinical trials.

■ Kava kava comes from the root of a plant in some Pacific islands. Used there for many generations and has been in Phase II and III clinical trials. It was available until recently as a complementary treatment but has been withdrawn due to concerns about hepatotoxicity.

References

Key references
Granville-Grossman KL, Turner P. The effect of propranolol on anxiety. Lancet 1966; i: 788–90
Klein DF. Delineation of two drug-responsive anxiety syndromes. Psychopharmacologia 1964; 5:397–408
Petursson H, Lader MH. Withdrawal from long-term benzodiazepine treatment. BMJ 1981; 283:643–5
Squires RF, Braestrup C. Benzodiazepine receptors in rat brain. Nature 1977; 274:732–4

Further reading
Cooper SJ. Anxiolytics, sedatives and hypnotics. In: Seminars in Clinical Psychopharmacology (King DJ, ed). London: Gaskell, 1995; pp 103–37 (second edition expected in 2004)
Griebel G. Is there a future for neuropeptide receptor ligands in the treatment of anxiety disorders? Pharmacol Therapeut 1999; 82:1–61 (Gives a comprehensive review of this field but is for the seriously enthusiastic only)
National Institute for Clinical Excellence Final Appraisal Determination. Zaleplon, zolpidem and zopiclone for the short-term management of insomnia. http://www.nice.org.uk
Paul SM. GABA and glycine. In: Psychopharmacology, the Fourth Generation of Progress (Bloom FE , Kupfer DJ, eds). New York: Raven Press, 1994; pp 87–94
Royal College of Psychiatrists. Benzodiazepines: risks, benefits or dependence. A re-evaluation. Council Report CR59. London: Royal College of Psychiatrists, 1997
Shiloh R, Nutt D, Weizman A. Atlas of Psychiatric Pharmacology. London: Martin Dunitz, 1999

7 Drugs of abuse

Why take drugs?

- For pleasure, to get a 'rush', euphoria, i.e. for positive reinforcement or reward.
- Anxiolytic or to overcome withdrawal, i.e. negative reinforcement.
- Because their use cannot be controlled, overwhelming urge, compulsion.

The faster the onset of the drug effects, the better the 'rush':

Slow				Fast
Chewing tobacco	$\rightarrow$		snuff	$\rightarrow$	cigarettes
Coca leaves	$\rightarrow$	coca paste	$\rightarrow$	cocaine	$\rightarrow$	crack cocaine
Methadone	$\rightarrow$	morphine	$\rightarrow$	snorted heroin	$\rightarrow$	intravenous heroin

History

- The pattern of drug use changes with time depending on what is available and how much it costs.
- Many drugs, which are now considered 'addictive', were often introduced for medical purposes.
- Alcohol:
  - Evidence of fermentation processes occurring approximately 7000 years ago.
  - Currently is the mostly widely used legal drug and relative cost is decreasing.
- Opioids:
  - Opium has been used medically since ancient times.
  - Morphine was isolated in 1805.

- – Methadone was first synthesised in Germany during World War II.
- ■ Stimulants:
  - – Amphetamine was synthesised in the late 1880s for therapeutic purposes.
  - – Cocaine alkaloid was first isolated in 1860 and used as a local anaesthetic.
  - – Methamphetamine (derivative of amphetamine) is increasingly used on the west coast of the USA and in some Asian countries.
- ■ Cannabis:
  - – Its effects have been documented for many centuries.
  - – Its nonmedical use, for its hedonic properties, began in the early 19th century in Europe.
- ■ Hallucinogens, include both natural (psilocybin) and synthetic (lysergic acid diethylamide, LSD) compounds:
  - – Hallucinogenic powers of LSD were discovered when it was accidentally absorbed in 1943. In the 1950s the term 'psychedelic' was coined.
  - – Use of psychedelic drugs predominated in the 1960s.
- ■ Tobacco, a native plant of the American continent:
  - – Believed to have been first used in the first century.
  - – Smoked in Europe from around the end of the 15th century.

In conceptualizing the recreational use/misuse of drugs, different models have been applied:
- ■ Medical (disease model).
- ■ Psychological (learning theory).
- ■ Philosophical/moral.

Legal issues (UK)

- ■ The Misuse of Drugs Act 1971 relates to the manufacture, supply and possession of 'Controlled Drugs'. Drugs are ascribed to one of three classes based on the perceived harmfulness when they are misused; the penalties are set accordingly. (See the British National Formulary, BNF, for the complete listing.)
  - – *Class A* includes cocaine, diamorphine (heroin), dipipanone, lysergide (LSD), methadone, methylenedioxymethamphetamine (MDMA or Ecstasy), morphine, opium, pethidine, phencyclidine and class B substances when prepared for injection.
  - – *Class B* includes oral amphetamines, barbiturates, codeine and pentazocine.

- *Class C* includes certain drugs related to the amphetamines such as benzfetamine and chlorphentermine, buprenorphine, diethylpropion, mazindol, meprobamate, pemoline, pipradrol, most benzodiazepines, androgenic and anabolic steroids, clenbuterol, cannabis and cannabis resin (controversially reclassified from Class B to C in 2004).
- See the BNF for regulations related to prescribing of controlled drugs.

Scientific background

Drugs of abuse and dopamine (DA)

- Drugs of abuse increase DA concentration in the nucleus accumbens of the mesolimbic system (see Fig. 1.3, p. 3, and Fig. 1.7, p. 11).
- Increase in DA function is key in mediating positive reinforcement:
  - DA increased by cocaine, amphetamine, alcohol, opiates, nicotine, cannabinoids.
  - Benzodiazepines (BDZs) are the only drugs of abuse not shown to significantly increase DA.
- Nucleus accumbens:
  - Has high levels of D_3 receptors.
  - DA release here, and in the amygdala, is also involved in learning associations, i.e. draws attention to certain significant events.
- Reduced DA concentrations are seen in withdrawal states and are likely to be associated with depression, irritability, dysphoria.
- Sensitisation (a progressive increase in an effect of a drug with repeated administration; see Chapter 2) is associated with stimulant abuse.
- DA is modulated by opioids (see Fig. 1.3, p. 3):
  - This is the pharmacological basis for naltrexone's efficacy in treatment of alcohol dependence.

Alcohol

Neuropharmacology

There is no 'alcohol receptor' as such. Alcohol primarily modulates ion channel function – GABA-BDZ, *N*-methyl D-aspartate (NMDA), 5-HT$_3$ receptors – and the following neurotransmitter systems are involved.

Alcohol and GABA function

■ Alcohol mediates many of its actions through modulating GABA function – it is an agonist at $GABA_A$ receptors (see Chapters 1 and 6 for details of GABA receptor).

■ Different subunits of the receptor confer different alcohol sensitivity. Recently α_5-containing receptors shown to be involved with alcohol reinforcement (see also Chapter 6).

■ This varied sensitivity is a possible mechanism of vulnerability to alcoholism.

■ Chronic ethanol exposure is associated with reduced GABA function and reduced levels of specific receptor subunits leading to tolerance.

Alcohol and glutamate function

■ Alcohol is an NMDA antagonist causing decreased Ca^{2+} influx into neurones and decreased excitability (see Fig. 1.14, p. 25).

■ Chronic ethanol exposure increases NMDA receptor function which:
  - may account for effects on memory, i.e. amnesia;
  - leads in withdrawal to a hyperexcitable state, which is probably the mechanism underlying seizures and brain damage.

Alcohol and monoamine function

Dopamine (DA)

■ Reduced DA responses are seen in patients with alcoholism.

■ These reduced responses may predict relapse and be associated with depressive symptomatology – dysphoria, irritability, restlessness.

■ Association reported in some groups with D_2 receptor polymorphism.

■ D_2 receptor-deficient mice show marked aversion to alcohol.

Noradrenaline (NA)

Increased activity may occur in alcohol withdrawal, however lofexidine (α_2 adrenoceptor agonist) does not symptomatically improve alcohol withdrawal.

Serotonin (5-HT)

■ Low levels of 5-HT particularly associated with type II alcoholism (early onset, high impulsivity, positive family history of alcoholism, male predominance):
  - increased 5-HT function may lead to craving.

■ High levels of 5-HT may be associated with type I alcoholism (later onset, mixed gender, anxious):

- increased 5-HT function may lead to anxiety.
■ 5-HT is implicated in many disorders which co-exist with alcoholism:
  - depression/suicide, anxiety disorders, bulimia nervosa.

Alcohol and other receptors

■ Opioids: see 'Scientific background' above.
■ Neuropeptide Y (NPY): there are many peptides which are proposed to be involved in addiction. NPY is the latest to attract attention.

Neurochemistry and neuropharmacology of treating alcohol withdrawal and dependence

Neurochemistry of alcohol withdrawal

Alcohol withdrawal is associated with:

■ Increased activity in:
  - NMDA receptor $\longrightarrow$ $\uparrow Ca^{2+}$ influx to cell
  - L-subtype of Ca^{2+} channel

    $\downarrow$

    Hyperexcitability
    and cell death

  - NA activity.
■ Decreases in:
  - GABA function.
  - Mg^{2+} inhibition of the NMDA receptor (see Fig. 1.14, p 25).
  - DA activity.

Treatment of alcohol withdrawal

■ BDZs to increase GABA function.
■ Vitamins (thiamin (B_1), B complex) as alcoholics are likely to be vitamin (especially thiamine) deficient due to poor diet and poor absorption. Parenteral thiamine preferable as poorly absorbed orally (caution as anaphylaxis is a rare but recognised risk).
■ Carbamazepine has shown efficacy and may be an alternative if BDZs contraindicated or ineffective.

Neurochemistry of alcohol dependence (Fig. 7.1)

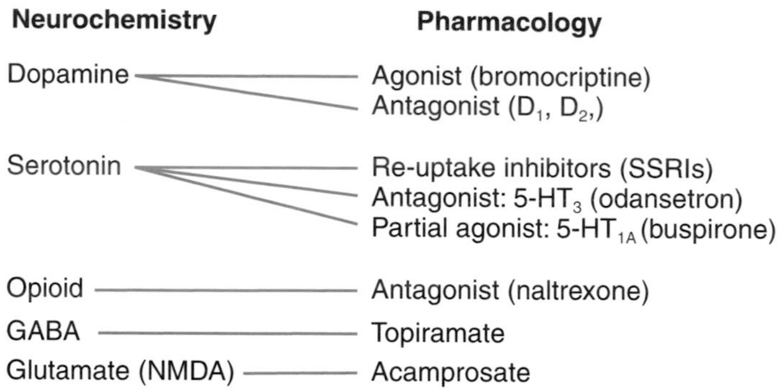

Neurochemistry
Pharmacology
Dopamine
Agonist (bromocriptine)
Antagonist (D_1, D_2,)
Serotonin
Re-uptake inhibitors (SSRIs)
Antagonist: 5-HT_3 (odansetron)
Partial agonist: 5-HT_{1A} (buspirone)
Opioid
Antagonist (naltrexone)
GABA
Topiramate
Glutamate (NMDA)
Acamprosate

Figure 7.1 *Neurochemistry related to drugs that have been used in the treatment of alcoholism.*

Treatment of alcohol dependence

- A variety of drugs have been used in the treatment of alcohol dependence with limited success.
- Comorbid psychiatric disorders may require treatment but patients should not be started on psychotropic drugs for two to three weeks as symptoms may subside spontaneously following abstinence.

Some specific drugs for alcohol dependence

Disulfiram

- Disulfiram inhibits aldehyde dehydrogenase (Fig. 7.2).
- This leads to a build-up of acetaldehyde if alcohol is consumed causing adverse effects:
  - Nausea and vomiting.
  - Flushing.

Alcohol
Alcohol dehydrogenase
Acetaldehyde
X
Aldehyde dehydrogenase (ALDH)
Acetate
Disulfiram

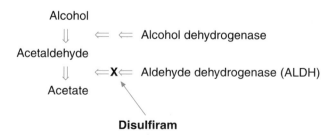

Figure 7.2 *Disulfiram inhibits the metabolism of acetaldehyde to acetate.*

- Palpitations.
- Headache.
- Hypotension.

■ Contraindications are psychosis, severe liver or cardiac disease, epilepsy.

■ Supervision or witnessed consumption is associated with improved outcome.

Acamprosate

■ Taurine derivative.

■ Its exact pharmacology is still not clear but it antagonises glutamate NMDA receptor function, possibly through effect on AMPA receptors.

■ Approximately doubles abstinence rates to about 20–40% and increases also 'time to first drink'.

■ Reduces likelihood of an episode of drinking becoming a relapse.

■ Adverse effects generally mild: gastrointestinal disturbance.

■ Contraindicated if severe liver damage.

■ Described as 'anticraving' – contentious.

■ Acamprosate may be more efficacious in 'anxious' people, though not supported in a recent review.

Naltrexone

■ Opioid antagonist (nonselective: μ, κ, δ receptors).

■ In alcohol dependence:
- reduces relapse rate;
- reduces craving.

■ Contraindicated in acute hepatitis or liver failure.

Topiramate

■ Anticonvulsant drug recently reported to improve drinking behaviour (reduced drinking days, greater abstinence rates) in alcohol-dependent subjects.

■ Given when still actively drinking but in an abstinence-focused treatment plan (other trials generally give drugs when abstinent).

Treatment of comorbidity

Depression

■ Depressive symptoms and disorder are common and as likely to precede alcohol abuse as to be a consequence of it.

■ Persistent depressive symptoms following withdrawal from alcohol should be treated (see Chapter 4).

■ Early trials of antidepressants in alcohol disorder and depression (TCAs and SSRIs) did not consistently show efficacy. However, more recent studies suggest SSRIs may improve drinking behaviour and depression in depressed alcoholics. There is evidence that use of SSRIs in nondepressed type II alcohol dependence either results in no improvement, or maybe worsens outcome.

Anxiety

■ As with depression, anxiety may be a cause and a consequence of alcohol abuse.

■ Panic attacks and generalised anxiety disorder (GAD) can emerge from alcohol dependence.

■ Treatment of comorbid anxiety disorders has not been studied to the same extent as for depression.

■ BDZs should rarely be used due to their addictive potential.

■ Buspirone has been shown to reduce anxiety and drinking behaviour.

■ Antidepressants have been shown to have some benefit in reducing panic attacks in alcoholics.

Schizophrenia

■ Fourfold increase of alcoholism in schizophrenia; more common than drug misuse.

■ Substance misuse leads to increased family conflict (high expressed emotion), a factor in schizophrenic relapse.

Opiates/opioids

The term 'opiates' refers to natural substances (e.g. morphine, codeine) and 'opioids' to semisynthetic (e.g. heroin, dihydrocodeine (DF118)) and synthetic (e.g. methadone) compounds.

Opioids

■ Act as agonists at:
  – μ (mu) receptors – analgesia, euphoria, positive reinforcement, respiratory depression;
  – κ (kappa) receptors – dysphoria, sedation.

■ Acute effects: miosis, euphoria, tranquillity, drowsiness, itching, nausea.

■ Chronic effects: anhedonia, depression, insomnia, dependence.

■ Mechanism of tolerance to opioids is not well understood with no clear changes in opiate receptor numbers reported, suggesting intracellular changes or alterations in other systems.

Opioid withdrawal

- Symptoms:
  - mydriasis, diarrhoea, dysphoria, insomnia, restlessness, 'craving';
  - associated with increased noradrenergic function: tachycardia, sweating, piloerection, rhinorrhoea, shivering.
- Opioid withdrawal is associated with increased NA function due to opioid effects in the locus coeruleus:
  - Acute effects of opioids are to inhibit cAMP and reduce NA neuronal firing.
  - With chronic exposure, compensatory upregulation of cAMP occurs, with an increase in NA tone which is revealed on withdrawal of opioids.
- Treatment:
  - Opioid substitute therapy.
  - Symptomatic treatment for gastrointestinal disturbance, insomnia, muscle aches.
  - Lofexidine, an α_2 agonist to reduce NA-related symptoms (side-effects: sedation, hypotension).

Substitute therapies in opioid addiction

Principle: use drugs with a longer half-life than 'street' opioids (Fig 7.3)

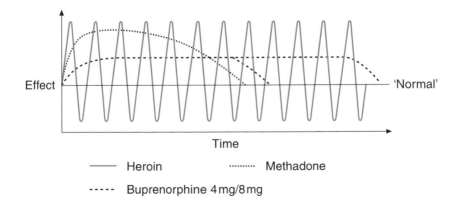

Figure 7.3 *Pharmacology of opioid substitute therapy. Methadone is a relatively long-acting full agonist and buprenorphine a long-acting partial agonist and their use avoids the 'highs' alternating with 'lows' associated with heroin.*

Methadone

- Full μ opiate agonist.
- $t_{1/2}$ = approx. 24 hours.
- Widely used in maintenance and detoxification.
- Levo-alpha-acetylmethadol (LAAM) (not licensed) is a congener of methadone and is a longer-acting alternative which can be given once every two to three days.

Buprenorphine

- Partial agonist at μ opiate receptor, leads to reduced risk of fatal respiratory depression.
- Antagonist at κ opiate receptor, which may be why buprenorphine is less likely to cause dysphoria.
- $t_{1/2}$ = >24 hours, so withdrawal syndrome less severe.
- Safer than full agonists and prevents the full effect of additional full (street) opiate agonists by antagonising its effects (see Chapter 2 for discussion about partial agonists).

Naltrexone

- Oral nonselective opioid antagonist – blocks acute opioid effects.
- Long-acting (active metabolite gives effective $t_{1/2}$ of 96 hours).
- Used to prevent relapse in drug-free subjects.
- Good compliance and monitoring associated with better outcome.
- Most common side-effects are gastrointestinal.

Stimulants

Cocaine

- 'Crack' is the free base of cocaine and can be smoked, inhaled or injected giving a faster rate of onset than cocaine (snorted).
- Cocaine inhibits DA (most important), 5-HT and NA re-uptake.
- Pharmacokinetics of delivery important: cocaine 'rush' intensity due to fast uptake.
- Acute effects: euphoria (related to DA transporter blockade), confusion, psychosis, ↑blood pressure/pulse (can result in stroke, seizure), formication, and then a 'crash' – see below.
- Chronic effects: paranoia, psychosis, anorexia, depression.
- Complex adaptation to chronic use: variable effect on D_1, D_2 receptor numbers/function.

- Withdrawal 'crash':
  - depression, anxiety, hypersomnia, anergia;
  - treatment with antidepressants (desipramine) is not thought to be effective in preventing this 'crash'.

Pharmacotherapy for cocaine addiction in development

- Vaccines.
- Partial D_3 agonist (in animal studies reduces response to cocaine cues).
- Drugs such as disulfiram and baclofen, and DA agonists such as bromocriptine, are also in trials.

Amfetamine

- Inhibits DA re-uptake and also stimulates DA release.
- Similar effects to cocaine.

Hallucinogens

Phencyclidine (PCP)

- Glutamate (NMDA) receptor antagonist.
- Acute effects:
  - delusions, paranoia, disordered thinking (schizophrenic like), illusions/hallucinations;
    ↑blood pressure/pulse.
- chronic: cognitive impairment, depression, weight loss.

Ketamine

- Glutamate (NMDA) receptor antagonist.
- Used as anaesthetic agent but is abused as a 'club drug'.
- Can be injected or snorted.
- Similar effects to PCP: prominent dissociative effects, dream-like states and hallucinations.

Lysergic acid diethylamide (LSD)

- Primary effect is via the serotonergic system (5-HT$_{2A}$ agonist).
- Acute effects ('trip'): mood swings, delusions, synaesthesia (e.g. hearing colours), panic, ↑ blood pressure/pulse.
- Later effects: 'flashbacks', reoccurrence of unpleasant acute effects.

Enactogens

Prototype: methylenedioxymethamfetamine (MDMA, Ecstasy):

■ Stimulant/hallucinogenic depending on contents of the tablet.
■ Derivatives: methylenedioxyamfetamine (MDA, Adam), methylenedioxyethylamfetamine (MDEA, Eve).
■ 5-HT neurotoxin (at dorsal raphe nucleus) leading to:
  – in animal studies: loss of 5-HT neurones, 5-HT transporters, ↓5-HIAA (5-HT metabolite) in CSF;
  – toxicity: MDA > MDMA > MDEA;
  – neurotoxicity of Ecstasy in humans is not clear.
■ Acute effects: empathy, ↑blood pressure/pulse, dehydration, renal/heart failure, ↑body temperature (greater with dancing), teeth clenching, ↓appetite.
■ After-effects: midweek blues/depression, disordered sleep.
■ Chronic effects: memory impairment, depression.
■ Use associated with flashbacks, psychosis, depression, anxiety.

Nicotine

■ Stimulant.
■ Primary site of action is the nicotinic ACh receptor.
■ Increases DA release in nucleus accumbens by increasing firing of ventral tegmental area DA neurones.
■ Tolerance is associated with receptor desensitisation and a compensatory upregulation of nicotinic receptors.
■ Receptor desensitisation can lessen overnight and hence the first cigarette of the day has the greatest effect.
■ Smoking associated with respiratory problems, lung cancer and cardiovascular disease.

Treatment of nicotine addiction

■ Various nicotine substitution regimens available:
  – inhalator is closest in pharmacokinetic profile to smoking;
■ Amfebutamone (bupropion):
  – DA and probable NA re-uptake inhibitor, which has been shown to aid smoking cessation.

Marijuana

Also known as cannabis, pot, weed, hash.

■ Main active chemical: δ-9-tetrahydrocannabinol (THC).

■ THC alters hippocampal and cerebellar neuronal activity.

■ Cannabinoid receptors located in nucleus accumbens.

■ May cause a dependence syndrome.

■ Acute effects: relaxation, time confusion, feeling of 'well-being', distorted perceptions, impairment of memory, concentration and co-ordination, ↑pulse, anxiety, psychosis (increasingly recognised as a precipitant of acute schizophrenic episodes).

■ Chronic effects: 'amotivational syndrome' – impaired attention, memory, learning, drive.

■ Smoking associated with respiratory problems, lung cancer and cardiovascular disease.

Benzodiazepines

These are discussed in Chapter 6.

References

Key references
Department of Health. Drug Misuse and Dependence – Guidelines on Clinical Management 1999. (Also known as Orange guidelines due to colour of cover.) http://www.doh.gov.uk/pub/docs/doh/dmfull.pdf
Iversen L. Cannabis and the brain. Brain 2003; 126:1252–70
Kessler RC, Crum RM, Warner LA *et al*. Lifetime co-occurrence of DSM-III-R alcohol abuse and dependence with other psychiatric disorders in the National Comorbidity Survey. Arch Gen Psychiatry 1997; 54:313–21
Kessler RC, McGonagle KA, Zhao S *et al*. Lifetime and 12-month prevalence of DSM-III-R psychiatric disorders in the United States. Arch Gen Psychiatry 1994; 51:8–19
Kreek MJ, LaForge KS, Butelman E. Pharmacotherapy of addictions. Nat Rev Drug Discov 2002; 1:710–26
Lingford-Hughes AR, Nutt D. The neurobiology of addiction and implications for treatment. Br J Psychiatry 2003; 182:97–100
Nutt DJ. Alcohol and the brain: pharmacological insights. Br J Psychiatry 1999; 175:114–19
Ward J, Hall W, Mattick RP. Role of maintenance treatment in opioid dependence. Lancet 1999; 353:221–6

Further reading
'Addiction is a brain disease, and it matters'. A series of articles in Science 1997; 278:45–70
Altman J, Everitt BJ, Glautier S *et al*. The biological, social and clinical bases of drug addiction: commentary and debate. Psychopharmacology 1996; 125:285–345

Ashton CH. Pharmacology and effects of cannabis: a brief review. Br J Psychiatry 2000; 178:101–6. (one of a series of articles about cannabis)

Berridge KC, Robinson TE. What is the role of dopamine in reward: hedonic impact, reward learning or incentive salience? Brain Res Rev 1998; 28:309–69

Di Chiara G. A motivational learning hypothesis of the role of mesolimbic dopamine in compulsive drug use. J Psychopharmacol 1998; 12:54–67

Dual Diagnosis. A series of articles in Addict Behav, 1998; vol. 23:717–946

Garbutt JC, West SL, Carey TS et al. Pharmacological treatment of alcohol dependence. JAMA 1999; 281:1318–25

Koob GF, Sanna PB, Bloom FE. Neuroscience of addiction. Neuron 1998; 21:467–76

Koob GF, Rocio M, Carrera A et al. Substance dependence as a compulsive behavior. J Psychopharmacol 1998; 12:39–48

Soyka M. Alcoholism and schizophrenia. Addiction 2000; 95:1613–18

8 Drug treatments for child and adolescent disorders

Background

- Increased clinical interest in child and adolescent psychopharmacology has outstripped research, with the exception of attention deficit/hyperactivity disorder (ADHD).
- This means there is generally a lack of an evidence base on which to base prescribing decisions.
- This is important as children are not simply 'mini adults':
  - Their developing brains almost certainly react differently to psychoactive medication.
  - Differences in metabolism make it likely that they will display different side-effect profiles to those seen in adults.

Attention deficit/hyperactivity disorder (ADHD)

Clinical background

- The DSM-IV diagnosis of ADHD consists of:
  - extremes of; *inattentive, impulsive* and *hyperactive* behaviour, which are
  - *pervasive,* of *early onset, unexplained* by other disorders and result in *impairment* and *disability.*
  - ICD-10 'hyperkinetic disorder' is more restrictive and requires more pervasive and impairing symptoms.
- Epidemiology of ADHD:
  - The prevalence is 3–8% (hyperkinetic disorder around 1.5%).
  - Three or four times more likely in boys than girls.
  - Highly comorbid – oppositional defiant disorder and conduct disorder most common.

- Only a small proportion of those with ADHD are identified, diagnosed and treated.
- ADHD is a chronic condition:
  - Commonly continues through adolescence and into adulthood.
  - If untreated is associated with educational and employment difficulties, relationship problems, increased accidents, substance misuse and delinquency.

Scientific background

Although the aetiology of ADHD is incompletely understood, increasing evidence supports a biological basis.

Genetic studies

- Heritability of ADHD estimated as greater than 0.8.
- Molecular genetics:
  - Replicated evidence implicating dopamine (DA) genes (D_4, D_5, the DA transporter).
  - Preliminary evidence implicating D_1 and $5-HT_{1B}$, DA-β-hydroxylase and SNAP-25 (involved in the regulation of neurotransmitter release).
  - Polygenic with small contribution from each gene (odds ratios: 1.2–1.9).

Brain imaging and electrophysiology

- Structural/functional abnormalities have been shown in frontal, temporal and parietal cortical regions, basal ganglia, callosal areas and cerebellum.
- Abnormalities evident early in development, nonprogressive and not a consequence of stimulant treatment.

Neuropsychology

- Studies demonstrate deficits in higher-order cognitive functions, including working memory and inhibition, motivational processes, memory, timing and time perception.

Neurotransmitters

Converging evidence for catecholamine dysregulation from:

- animal models;
- molecular genetic findings;
- functional imaging studies;
- the effectiveness of stimulants (related to DA) and noradrenaline (NA) drugs in treatment.

Management of ADHD

■ Multimodal intervention is usually indicated and should target both the core ADHD symptoms and associated or comorbid problems.

■ Psychological interventions, educational change, medication and diet should all be available, and their use should be guided by an individualised treatment plan.

Non-pharmacological treatments

■ Psychoeducational measures:
  – Education and advice should be the base of any treatment offered.

■ Parent training and behavioural interventions in the family:
  – Effectiveness shown in randomised controlled trials (RCTs).
  – There are many approaches, and evidence-based treatment manuals are available.

■ Behavioural interventions (preschool or school):
  – Effective in reducing hyperactive behaviour and promoting social adjustment.
  – No one scheme has been shown to be superior to others.

Pharmacological treatments

Stimulant drugs

Used to treat ADHD symptoms since 1937.

Methylphenidate and dexamfetamine

■ Mechanism of action (see also Chapter 1):
  – Methylphenidate is a DA transporter blocker.
  – Dexamfetamine blocks the DA transporter and stimulates synaptic DA release.
  – Both drugs increase DA levels in the nucleus accumbens and therefore have abuse potential. However, the best available evidence suggests that treatment of ADHD with stimulants reduces rather than increases the likelihood of later substance misuse.

■ The pharmacokinetic, pharmacodynamic and clinical effects of both drugs are very similar:
  – Short half-life ($t_{1/2}$ = 3 hours), rapid onset of action (t_{max} = 1.5 hours) and short duration of action (3–4 hours).
  – Immediate release forms require multiple daily dosing (two or three times per day).

- – Extended-release preparations are becoming available with increased duration of action (8–12 hours depending on preparation). Currently (2004), one methylphenidate extended-release preparation using an osmotic pump system (OROS®) is available in the UK as of early 2004 (Concerta XL®).

■ Efficacy:
- – Short-term efficacy and effectiveness at reducing core ADHD symptoms established in a large number of clinical trials and meta-analyses (effect size approx. 0.7–1.0). Effective in around 70% of cases with around 95% having a clinically meaningful response to one drug or the other.
- – Effective – occurs after first dose.
- – Evidence for longer-term efficacy is much weaker as there are no truly long-term trials of stimulant treatment of ADHD.

■ Side-effects:
- – Most common: decreased appetite and insomnia (dose related).
- – Less common: depression, irritability, increase in tics and raised blood pressure.
- – Methylphenidate: rash and allergic reactions, blood dyscrasias and hepatotoxicity.

■ Monitoring of blood pressure and periodic full blood count, differential and platelets (methylphenidate) recommended.

■ Drug interactions (Table 8.1).

Table 8.1 *Selected drug interactions with stimulant drugs*

Action/effect	Drug/drug class
Inhibition of metabolism/increased plasma concentration of named drug	TCAs
	SSRIs
	Some anticonvulsants (phenobarbital, phenytoin, primidone)
Decreased therapeutic effect of named drugs	Antipsychotics
	Adrenergic neurone blockers (antihypertensive action)
Hypertension	MAOIs
	Oxytocin
	Doxapram
Increased plasma concentration of methylphenidate	Some anticonvulsants (phenobarbital, phenytoin, primidone)
?Sudden death (causal link not established)	Clonidine

■ Prescribing issues
- Despite continuing public and media controversy there is little evidence that methylphenidate or dexamphetamine are associated with any negative long-term treatment outcomes in ADHD.
- Large inter-individual variation requires wide dose titration to achieve balance between symptom reduction and side-effects.
- The requirement to take medication three times a day, and during school, can lead to practical and compliance problems, stigma, restriction in activities. Extended-release stimulant preparations may reduce some of these problems.
- The decision as to whether stimulant medication should be started will depend on the presentation of each individual case (Box 8.1).

Box 8.1 *Factors to consider before prescribing stimulants for ADHD*

Diagnosis of ADHD with severe core symptoms required

Are symptoms pervasive across all situations? If not, psychosocial interventions specific to situation should be given

Unless urgent need, consider psychosocial intervention first and only prescribe stimulants after reasonable failed trial (e.g. three months)

Age:
■ Preschool children: methylphenidate not licensed below six years of age; evidence for efficacy of stimulants less secure
■ Adolescents: possible lower response rates, problems with compliance and increased risk of drug misuse
■ Adults: less evidence for efficacy of stimulants, lower response rate, increased risk of drug misuse, TCAs probably first line

Attitudes of patient and carers to drug treatment

■ Guidance
- In the UK, the Scottish Intercollegiate Guidelines Network (SIGN) and the National Institute for Clinical Excellence (NICE) regard methylphenidate and dexamfetamine as a first-line treatment of ADHD. This is subject to diagnosis, initiation and management carried out by specialists in ADHD within a shared care protocol with primary care with at least six-monthly monitoring.

- The influential Multimodal Treatment Study of ADHD (MTA study) demonstrated the superiority of a carefully managed and structured medication package over both behavioural treatment and unstructured community-based pharmacological treatment. Components included more intensive medication regime, blind initial dose titration, supportive counselling and reading materials, and monthly consultations for dose adjustment.

Pemoline
- A longer-acting stimulant with main actions due to inhibition of DA reuptake.
- Comparable effectiveness to methylphenidate and dexamfetamine.
- UK licence for ADHD withdrawn due to severe liver toxicity in a number of patients.

Adderall XR®
- An extended-release mixed amfetamine salt preparation containing 25% levoamfetamine and 75% dextroamfetamine.
- Efficacy demonstrated for the treatment of ADHD symptoms in several RCTs.
- May have a small but statistically significant efficacy advantage over immediate-release methylphenidate. Adderall appears to have a longer duration of action than immediate-release methylphenidate from comparative studies.
- Licensed for the treatment of ADHD in the USA but not in the UK.

Nonstimulant drugs
Only atomoxetine is licensed for use in ADHD in the UK.

Tricyclic antidepressants (TCAs)
- Currently recommended in the UK as third-line treatment for ADHD, following unsuccessful and/or poorly tolerated trials of stimulants.
- TCAs are associated with a wide range of side-effects and are toxic in overdose (see Chapter 4) and should be used with extreme caution in children and adolescents.
- In terms of efficacy a systematic review concluded that:
  - Studies comparing stimulants with TCAs had many limitations.
  - Desipramine is more effective than placebo (withdrawn from the market in the UK due to concerns over cardiotoxicity).

- Imipramine shows inconsistent results and present insufficient data on which to base judgements.

Atomoxetine

■ A highly specific NA re-uptake inhibitor.

■ It affects DA as well as NA function and it is likely that clinical effects are associated with both effects.

■ No alteration of DA levels in the nucleus accumbens; thus is unlikely to be associated with abuse potential.

■ Metabolised by hepatic CYP-2D6 but no association between poor metaboliser status and increased adverse events reported.

■ All published industry-sponsored placebo-controlled RCTs in ADHD – four in children and adolescents (combined N = 759) and three in adults – reported atomoxetine superior to placebo in reduction of core ADHD symptoms (effect size: 0.6–0.8).

■ Few data currently available directly comparing atomoxetine and stimulant medications.

■ Although plasma $t_{1/2}$ of atomoxetine is short (approx. four hours) the behavioural effects last longer than predicted from the pharmacokinetics and once-daily dosing is effective.

■ Effects may be seen early but take two to four weeks to maximise.

■ Main side-effects are decreased appetite, vomiting, nausea, dizziness, asthenia and dyspepsia.

Other nonstimulant preparations
The following have been used in treating ADHD but there are insuffient data to assess efficacy:

■ Clonidine.

■ Bupropion.

■ Guanfacine.

■ Venlafaxine (contraindicated in children and adolescents).

Autism

Background

■ Autism is a pervasive developmental disorder consisting of qualitative impairment of social functioning, communication and restricted, repetitive and stereotyped patterns of behaviour and interests.

- Our understanding of its complex aetiology remains incomplete but there is evidence for reduced 5-HT neurotransmission and altered DA neurotransmission.
- Educational and behavioural treatments remain the mainstay of treatment for children and adolescents with autism.

Drug treatments for autism

There is increased interest in the role of medication as an adjunctive therapy for specific troublesome behaviours (rather than core symptoms), namely hyperactivity, aggression, withdrawal and repetitive, ritualized, stereotyped or self-injurious behaviours.

Antidepressants

Drugs primarily affecting 5-HT neurotransmission may show efficacy:
- Clomipramine has been demonstrated to be superior to placebo and desipramine on ratings of autistic symptoms (including stereotypies), anger and compulsive, ritualised behaviours.
- Adverse events associated with clomipramine, including QTc prolongation, tachycardia and seizures, mean it must be used with great care in this population.
- Fluvoxamine was superior to placebo in one study in reducing repetitive thoughts and behaviour, maladaptive behaviour and aggression. It also improved some aspects of social relatedness, particularly language use. However, another RCT has reported no difference between fluvoxamine and placebo.

Antipsychotics

Critics of the use of antipsychotics in children with autism suggest that they are being used merely as 'chemical strait-jackets' but this does not seem to be the case.

Typical antipsychotics (DA antagonists)
- Haloperidol has been the most intensely studied and remains the most established psychopharmacologic agent for children and adolescents with autism.
- Several RCTs have demonstrated haloperidol to be effective in reducing a wide range of maladaptive behaviours in children and adolescents with autism including hyperactivity, withdrawal, aggression and temper tantrums, stereotypies, mood lability, increased social relatedness and increased discriminant learning.

■ These positive effects need to be balanced against the frequent and disabling adverse reactions:
  - Short-term: excessive sedation and extrapyramidal side-effects are common.
  - Approximately one-third of children suffer from withdrawal dyskinesias and around 10% may develop tardive dyskinesia.
■ As a result, despite their proven effectiveness, many clinicians remain wary about using haloperidol in autism.

Atypical antipsychotics (combined DA and 5-HT antagonists)
■ There are published reports of risperidone, olanzapine and quetiapine in the treatment of autism.
■ They seem to be effective and well tolerated for the treatment of tantrums, aggression and self-injurious behaviour.
■ Increased appetite and weight gain, fatigue, drowsiness, dizziness and drooling were common with risperidone.
■ Relatively small doses appear effective and seem independent of common adverse events such as drowsiness and fatigue.

Depressive disorders

■ Psychotherapeutic interventions, particularly cognitive behavioural therapy (CBT) and interpersonal therapy (IPT) are effective in the treatment of many children and adolescents with depressive symptoms and mild-to-moderate depressive episodes and should probably be considered first-line treatment.
■ See Chapter 4 for details of antidepressants.

Tricyclic antidepressants
■ TCAs are of unlikely benefit in the treatment of depression in prepubertal children.
■ There is marginal evidence to support the use of TCAs in the treatment of depression in adolescents but benefits are likely to be moderate at best.
■ Side-effects and toxicity in overdose mean extreme caution is required in their use.

Selective serotonin re-uptake inhibitors (SSRIs)
■ There has been a rapid increase in the use of SSRIs in children and adolescents, which has outstripped the evidence base.

■ There has been recent concern from unpublished data in industry-sponsored trials of SSRIs in child and adolescent depression suggesting that these drugs may lead to an increased rate of suicidal ideation. This prompted a review of their use by the UK Committee on Safety of Medicines (CSM) in 2003, which ruled that for major depressive disorder (MDD) in children and adolescents under the age of 18:

  – Paroxetine, sertraline, citalopram and escitalopram, fluvoxamine and venlafaxine are contraindicated on the basis of unfavourable or unassessable balance of risks and benefits.

  – The balance of risks and benefits for fluoxetine appears to be favourable and it can still be used.

■ There is, as yet, no guidance on how to treat those under 18 years of age with MDD who fail to respond to an adequate psychosocial intervention and fluoxetine.

Manic episodes and bipolar affective disorder (BD)

■ There is considerable confusion and disagreement over the most appropriate ways in which to diagnose manic episodes and BD in child and adolescent populations.

■ In the UK a diagnosis of BD is still rarely made (it is much more common in the USA).

■ It is very difficult to know exactly which patients have been included in clinical trials for the treatment of early-onset BD and how to translate this into clinical practice.

■ Nevertheless it does seem to be the case that true manic episodes are difficult to modify without medication.

■ There is some evidence from case series and open-label trials for the efficacy of lithium, valproate/valproate semisodium and carbamazepine in the treatment of early-onset mania.

■ A small RCT showed that adding quetiapine to valproate is more effective than valproate alone for the treatment of mania in adolescents.

Obsessive–compulsive disorder (OCD)

■ The SSRIs sertraline and fluvoxamine have both been demonstrated to be safe and effective treatments for paediatric OCD and are licensed for use in children and adolescents in the UK.

■ Long-term treatment is well tolerated and effective at maintaining improvement with continued improvement for up to one year.

■ Obsessional symptoms may relapse on discontinuation of treatment but it is suggested that withdrawal of treatment should be attempted after 1–1½ years and restarted if significant symptoms reoccur.

■ Paediatric OCD may not respond as well to some SSRIs as adult OCD:
  – 20–25% are symptom free at the end of a course of treatment, 20–50% have some improvement and about 25% show no improvement.

Anxiety disorders

■ The use of drug treatments in the management of child and adolescent anxiety disorders remains contentious with many clinicians arguing that these disorders are most appropriately treated with psychosocial interventions.

■ However, success rates for cognitive behavioural psychotherapy are 70–80% so significant numbers of children require further intervention.

Benzodiazepines

Generally efficacious, however adverse events and risk of tolerance mean that they should only be considered when other pharmacological approaches have failed and should only be prescribed for very short periods of time.

Tricyclic antidepressants (TCAs)

RCTs of TCAs conducted in paediatric anxiety have not demonstrated clear efficacy and they should not be considered as first-line treatments for these disorders.

Selective serotonin re-uptake inhibitors (SSRIs)

■ Both fluvoxamine and sertraline have been reported in short-term RCTs to be efficacious in paediatric generalised anxiety disorder.

■ Neither drug is licensed in this age group for this indication. In view of the recent decision to exclude their use in paediatric MDD, but to continue their use in paediatric OCD, it is not clear what the current status of guidance is for their prescription in anxiety disorders.

References

Key references
Emslie GJ, Rush AJ, Weinberg WA *et al*. A double-blind, randomized, placebo-controlled trial of fluoxetine in children and adolescents with depression. Arch Gen Psychiatry 1997; 54:1031–7

Hazell P, O'Connell D, Heathcote D, Henry D. Tricyclic drugs for depression in children and adolescents. (Cochrane Review). In: The Cochrane Library, Issue 1, 2004.

James AC, Javaloyes AM. The treatment of bipolar disorder in children and adolescents. J Child Psychol Psychiatry All Disciplines 2001; 42:439–49

McCracken JT, McGough J, Shah B *et al*. Risperidone in children with autism and serious behavioral problems. N Engl J Med 2002; 347:314–21

MTA Co-operative Group. A 14-month randomized clinical trial of treatment strategies for attention-deficit/hyperactivity disorder. The MTA Co-operative Group. Multimodal Treatment Study of Children with ADHD. Arch Gen Psychiatry 1999; 56:1073–86

Riddle MA, Reeve EA, Yaryura-Tobias JA *et al*. Fluvoxamine for children and adolescents with obsessive-compulsive disorder: a randomized, controlled, multicenter trial. J Am Acad Child Adolesc Psychiatry 2001; 40:222–9

Further reading
British Association for Psychopharmacology. Child and learning disability psychopharmacology. J Psychopharmacol 1997; 11(4):291–4.

Child Adolesc Psychiatric Clin N Am 2000; 9(1): Psychopharmacology. (An entire volume devoted to the North American perspective on child and adolescent psychopharmacology)

Eur Child Adolesc Psychiatry 2000; 9(Suppl. 1) (This complete supplement comprises a series of excellent reviews on child and adolescent psychopharmacology).

Greenhill LL, Pliszka S, Dulcan MK *et al*. for the American Academy of Child and Adolescent Psychiatry. Practice parameter for the use of stimulant medications in the treatment of children, adolescents, and adults. J Am Acad Child Adolesc Psychiatry 2001; 41:26S–49S

Hill P, Taylor E. An auditable protocol for treating attention deficit/hyperactivity disorder. Arch Dis Childhood 2001; 84:404–9

MTA Co-operative Group. Moderators and mediators of treatment response for children with attention-deficit/hyperactivity disorder. The Multimodal Treatment Study of children with ADHD. Arch Gen Psychiatry 1999; 56:1088–96

National Institute for Clinical Excellence Technology Appraisal Guidance No. 13. Guidance on the use of methylphenidate (Ritalin, Equasym) for Attention Deficit/Hyperactivity Disorder (ADHD) in childhood 2000. http://www.nice.org.uk

Solanto MV, Arnsten AF, Castellanos FX. Stimulant Drugs and ADHD: Basic and Clinical Neuroscience. New York: Oxford University Press, 2001

Volkow ND, Swanson JM. Variables that affect the clinical use and abuse of methylphenidate in the treatment of ADHD. Am J Psychiatry 2003; 160:1909–18

9 Drugs for dementia

Types of dementia

- Two main types of symptoms require treatment in the dementias:
  - Cognitive deficits (ranging from mild to severe).
  - Noncognitive features (behavioural and psychiatric symptoms of dementia, BPSD, consisting of affective, psychotic and behavioural disturbances).
- Types of dementia relevant to treatment:
  - Alzheimer's disease (AD).
  - Dementia with Lewy bodies (commonly have motor features of Parkinson's disease).
  - Vascular dementia (multi-infarct dementia, small vessel dementia, infarcts of strategic areas).

History

- The cholinergic hypothesis of AD led to initial studies of acetylcholine (ACh) precursors lecithin and choline with little benefit.
- Anticholinesterase inhibitors:
  - tetrahydroaminoacridine (tacrine, THA) originally developed as an antiseptic in the 1940s and then used as a respiratory stimulant to reverse anaesthesia in the UK and Australia. First tested in AD in the 1980s, licensed in the USA;
  - donepezil, rivastigmine and galantamine licensed in the UK;
  - subject of Clinical Practice Guideline from the UK National Institute for Clinical Excellence (NICE) in 2001.
- Glutamate antagonist (memantine):
  - introduced in Germany in 1982 for organic brain syndromes;
  - licensed in Europe in 2002 for AD.

Scientific background

Alzheimer's disease

Figure 9.1 outlines risk factors and pathology of AD.

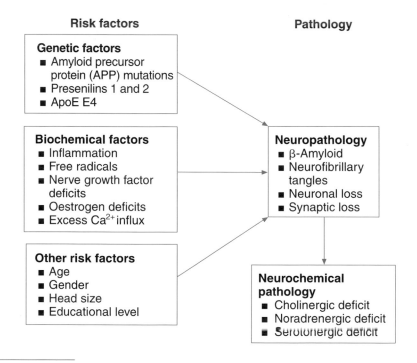

Figure 9.1 *Risk factors and pathology of Alzheimer's disease.*

Targets for drug intervention

■ Potential future intervention at level of genes, nerve growth factors, neuropathological changes.

■ Inflammation/neuroprotection:
  – Chronic nonsteroidal anti-inflammatory drugs (NSAIDs) decrease risk of AD by two to four times.
  – Oestrogen delays the onset of AD. Possible mechanisms include reversal of glucocorticoid damage, increased cerebral blood flow, prevention of neuronal atrophy, synergistic action with nerve growth factors.
  – Regular vitamin supplements (C or E) in the elderly associated with a lower risk of developing AD, possibly by reducing oxidative stress.

■ Neurochemistry (see below).

Cholinergic hypothesis of AD

Figure 9.2 outlines the main metabolic pathways of ACh.

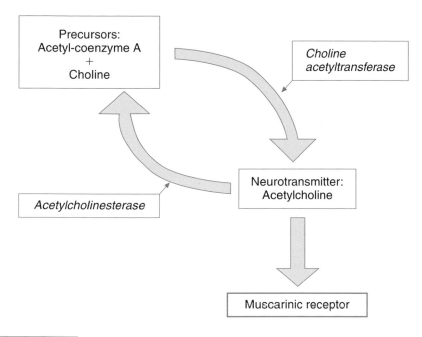

Figure 9.2 *The metabolic pathway of acetylcholine production and removal (see also Chapter 1).*

■ Antimuscarinic drugs (e.g. scopolamine) induce memory deficits and confusion in normal subjects.
■ In AD:
  – Substantial loss of cholinergic neurones in nucleus basalis (of Meynert), origin of cholinergic pathway projecting to all cortical areas and part of thalamus.
  – Post-mortem estimates of cholinergic function correlate with mental test scores, and amyloid plaque counts.
  – Reduced choline acetyltransferase, choline uptake and ACh release in neocortex.
■ Two cholinesterases present: acetylcholinesterase and butyrylcholinesterase (previously known as pseudocholinesterase).
  – Acetylcholinesterase found in cholinergic synapses in CNS and periphery.
  – Butyrylcholinesterase synthesised in liver and secreted into plasma. Also present in glial cells. Inhibition may lead to unwanted peripheral side-effects.

Monoamine deficits in AD

May account for behavioural changes in AD.

■ NA reduced especially in temporal cortex: loss of noradrenergic neurones and MAO are associated with depressive symptoms, also may relate to deficits in attention. Relative preservation of NA activity has been associated with delusions.

■ 5-HT function loss present in later stages: may relate to aggression, mood change.

■ DA, GABA and somatostatin concentrations not significantly changed.

Mechanism of neuronal damage in AD

Probably several mechanisms for neuronal damage in AD.

■ Influx of Ca^{2+} ions facilitated by glutamate causes neuronal death.

■ Prevention or reduction of this influx may be neuroprotective.

■ Blockade of NMDA receptor may achieve this.

Dementia with Lewy bodies

■ Greater cholinergic impairment than in AD correlated with visual hallucinations.

■ Relative preservation of muscarinic M_1 receptors.

■ May respond to procholinergic treatment. Noncognitive symptoms (especially visual hallucinations) may respond better than cognitive symptoms.

Vascular dementia

■ Vascular pathology is target for treatment.

■ Control of hypertension and diabetes are effective in prevention.

Assessment of outcome in clinical trials

Assessment is difficult and interpretation may be problematic; prevention of deterioration is important as well as improvement.

Cognitive performance

■ Alzheimer's Disease Assessment Scale (ADAS-cog): tests multiple areas of cognitive decline. Error score 0–70. Low score = high performance. Usually a primary outcome variable.

■ Mini-Mental State Examination (MMSE): screening instrument briefly tests several areas of cognition but not in depth. Score 0 (low performance) to 30 (high performance).

■ Numerous others, e.g. Abbreviated Mental Test Score (AMTS).

Global outcome measures
■ Clinicians Interview Based Impression of Change (CIBIC): interview-based assessment of global functioning. Score 1 (very much improved) to 7 (very much worse). CIBIC-plus includes interview with carer. Usually a primary outcome variable.
■ Clinical Dementia Rating (CDR) six domains rating deterioration in ability. Score 0 to 3 (severe).

Functional ability/activities of daily living (ADL)
■ Instrumental Activities of Daily Living (IADL): ability on household tasks, slightly adjusted for gender.
■ Interview for Deterioration in Daily living in Dementia (IDDD): deterioration in simple and more complex areas of daily living activity.

Behaviour and mood
■ Neuropsychiatric Inventory (NPI): psychiatric and behavioural changes in 12 domains.
■ Manchester and Oxford Universities Scale for the Psychopathological Assessment of Dementia (MOUSEPAD): semistructured interview of psychopathological and behavioural changes. Rates frequency only.

Individual drug classes

Cholinergic precursors
■ Precursor loading with choline or lecithin.
■ Ineffective.
■ Side-effect of rotting fish smell with choline.

Cholinesterase inhibitors

General issues
■ Potentiation of remaining cholinergic function so potential benefit related to amount of remaining cholinergic function.
■ Efficacy: most effective in early stages of dementia and lost as dementia progresses.
■ Dose-related gastrointestinal side-effects.

- Rarer adverse effects: stomach ulcers, sino-atrial block and atrioventricular block, seizures, transient ischaemic attacks.
- Interactions:
  - Cholinesterase inhibitors antagonised by procainamide, quinidine, aminoglycosides, antimuscarinic drugs.
  - Drugs used in anaesthesia: depolarising muscle relaxants (e.g. suxamethonium) may be potentiated; nondepolarising muscle relaxants (e.g. pancuronium) may be antagonised.
  - Galantamine metabolism reduced by some cytochrome P450 inhibitors (e.g. paroxetine, ketoconazole, erythromycin) leading to increased plasma concentrations.

Prescribing issues

Funding/implementation issues led to variable availability in the UK. Subject of national guideline from National Institute for Clinical Excellence (NICE) requiring availability of licensed anticholinesterases (donepezil, rivastigmine, galantamine) subject to specific requirements:

- Diagnosis of AD made in specialist clinic according to standard diagnostic criteria.
- Likelihood of compliance assessed.
- Tests required of cognitive, global, behavioural functioning and ADL before prescribing a drug.
- Initiation and maintenance prescription only if MMSE >12.
- Initial prescription only by specialists and transferred to general practitioners only recommended if agreed shared care protocol and agreed endpoints.
- Reassessment of progress after two to four months and drug continued only if global improvement together with cognitive improvement or lack of decline.
- Reassessment every six months if drug continued.

Tacrine (tetrahydroaminoacridine, THA), velnacrine

- Reversible acetylcholinesterase inhibitor; velnacrine is a derivative of THA.
- Several studies report THA significantly improves ADAS-cog, CIBIC and MMSE scores.
- Dose-dependent hepatic toxicity.
- THA licensed in the USA and France but not in the UK. No licence for velnacrine.

Metrifonate

- Originally developed to treat parasitic worms (schistosomiasis).
- Modest improvements in ADAS-cog, CIBIC. Inconsistent results with secondary variables.
- Generally well tolerated, side-effects mainly gastrointestinal and muscle weakness.
- Not licensed.

Donepezil

- Piperidine derivative, reversible cholinesterase inhibitor with high specificity for acetylcholinesterase over butyrylcholinesterase (may reduce peripheral side-effects).
- Long elimination half-life (70–80 hours) allows once-daily dosage.
- Metabolised by liver, not associated with hepatic toxicity.
- *Efficacy*: three systematic reviews, five randomised controlled trials:
  - improves CIBIC (cf. decline with placebo);
  - dose response on ADAS-cog up to 10 mg/day;
  - improvements over baseline decline with time as the disease progresses;
  - no significant improvement in quality of life (QoL) measures.
- Licensed in the UK.

Rivastigmine

- Carbamate derivative, reversible cholinesterase inhibitor.
- Rapidly absorbed; best taken with food to improve tolerability.
- Short elimination half-life <2 hours requires twice-daily dosage.
- Metabolised by cholinesterases, predominantly in liver.
- *Efficacy*: three systematic reviews, five randomised controlled trials:
  - improves global outcome measures compared with placebo;
  - inconsistent effect and dose response on cognitive measures;
  - significant improvement in QoL measures in one trial only.
- Licensed in the UK.

Galantamine

- Tertiary alkaloid, reversible acetylcholinesterase inhibitor, also potentiates the action of ACh at nicotinic receptors.
- Well-absorbed orally with low protein binding.
- Short elimination half-life (7 hours). Twice-daily dosage.
- Metabolised by cytochrome P450-2D6 and 3A4 with no significant active metabolites.

■ *Efficacy*: three systematic reviews, five randomised controlled trials:
  – improves CIBIC compared with placebo;
  – dose response improvements in ADAS-cog scores;
  – improvements in ADL at six months;
  – improvements in QoL measures at six months.
■ Licensed in the UK.

Glutamate antagonist

Memantine

■ Low–moderate, noncompetitive NMDA antagonist.
■ Elimination half-life 60–80 hours.
■ Limited trial evidence; benefits also limited.
■ Less marked deterioration in active group, greater retention of ADL skills.
■ Side-effects of hallucinations, confusion.
■ Awaiting NICE evaluation (expected 2005); currently patchy prescribing in the UK as a result.

Nootropics

■ Examples are piracetam, pramiracetam, oxiracetam.
■ Improve memory in animal models by unknown mechanism, possibly metabolic enhancement.
■ Limited evidence of improvement in patients with dementia.

Hormone replacement therapy (HRT)

■ Potential benefits suggested by epidemiological data.
■ Meta-analysis of five trials showed a limited positive effect from low-dose replacement (1.3 MMSE point gain after two months).
■ Also report of reduction in behavioural and psychiatric symptoms of dementia with HRT.
■ Ongoing controlled trials.
■ Risk–benefit needs evaluation in light of current concerns about increased risk of breast cancer and stroke with long-term HRT.

Drugs for vascular dementia

■ Salicylate: inhibits platelet cyclo-oxygenase and reduces platelet stickiness. Aspirin shown to improve cognition.
■ Cholinesterases:
  – modest improvements in six-month controlled trial;
  – as well tolerated in vascular dementia as in AD;
  – possible use in combination with memantine in the future.

- Ca^{2+} antagonists: nimodipine. Final common pathway in cell death is increase in intracellular calcium. Potential use in small vessel dementia.
- Improved red blood cell deformability thereby enhancing oxygen delivery, e.g. pentoxyphylline. May be effective in large vessel dementia.
- Propentofylline, a xanthine derivative, protects against cell damage by increasing extracellular adenosine. This reduces the damaging activation of microglia. Preliminary results promising.
- Vasodilators, e.g. cyclandelate, papaverine, cinnarizine. Ineffective.
- Ergot derivatives. Mechanism unknown. Very modest improvements compared to placebo.
- Ginkgo biloba – reported to decrease platelet aggregation and blood viscosity through unknown mechanism. Effective in controlled studies. Side-effects include subarachnoid or subdural haemorrhage.

Treatment of behavioural and psychiatric symptoms of dementia (BPSD)

Principles
- Careful definition of symptoms with elimination/treatment of physical causes, e.g infections, cardiovascular disease, constipation.
- Optimise the personal and physical environment, consider psychosocial factors and educate carers.
- Avoid/minimise drug causes, e.g. antimuscarinic (worsen cognition), anti-adrenergic (postural hypotension) and long elimination half-life drugs.

Depressive symptoms/disorders
- Common but underdiagnosed and undertreated.
- Few treatment studies: antidepressants may be useful. SSRIs probably preferred over older TCAs.
- Review and consider stopping antidepressant after 6–12 months; depression often goes as dementia progresses.

Psychotic symptoms
- More common in AD than vascular dementia.
- Typical antipsychotics have been traditional treatment with no evidence that any one is more effective than others. Extrapyramidal side-effects (EPSEs) especially in dementia with Lewy bodies.

■ Atypical antipsychotics have been increasingly used: fewer EPSEs and less cognitive impairment than typicals. Long-term safety not proven.

– The Committee on Safety of Medicines (CSM) in the UK has recently (2004) issued a warning of increased risk of cerebrovascular adverse events in elderly patients taking olanzapine and risperidone. The risk is especially raised in those with pre-existing cerebrovascular disease. The mechanism, and risk with other antipsychotics, is unclear.

■ Plan to stop treatment after three to nine months as psychosis often goes as dementia progresses.

Agitation/aggression
Antipsychotic drugs are mainstay of treatment (see previous section for issues in prescribing).

References

Key references
Bowen DM, Smith CB, White P, Davidson AN. Neurotransmitter-related enzymes and indices of hypoxia in senile dementia and other abiotrophies. Brain 1976; 99:459–96
Perry EK, Tomlinson BE, Blessed G *et al*. Correlation of cholinergic abnormalities with senile plaques and mental test scores in senile dementia. BMJ 1978; ii:1457–9
Schneider LS, Pollock VE, Lyness SA. A meta-analysis of controlled trials of neuroleptic treatment in dementia. J Am Geriatr Soc 1990; 38:553–63.
Wolfson C, Moride Y, Perrault A *et al*. Drug treatments for Alzheimer's disease. 1. Comparative analysis of clinical trials. Canadian Coordinating Office for Health Technology Assessment (CCOHTA), Ottawa, 2000

Further reading
Allen NHP, Burns AB. The non-cognitive features of dementia. Rev Clin Ger 1995; 5:57–75
Alzheimer A. On certain peculiar disease of old age. Hist Psychiatry 1991; ii:71–101
Bryson HM, Benfield P. Donepezil. Drugs Aging 1997; 10:234–9.
Clegg A, Bryant J, Nicholson T *et al*. Clinical and cost-effectiveness of donepezil, rivastigmine and galantamine for Alzheimer's disease. Health Technology Assessment report on behalf of the National Institute for Clinical Excellence (2000). http://www.nice.org.uk
Forette F, Seux M-L, Staessen JA *et al*. Prevention of dementia in randomised double-blind placebo-controlled systolic hypertension in Europe (Syst-Eur) trial. Lancet 1998; 351:1347–51
Morris MC, Beckett LA, Scherr PA *et al*. Vitamin E and vitamin C supplement use and risk of incident Alzheimer disease. Alzheimer Dis Assoc Disord 1998; 12:121–6
National Institute for Clinical Excellence Technology Appraisal Guidance No. 19. Guidance on the use of donepezil, rivastigmine and galantamine for the treatment of Alzheimer's disease, 2001. http://www.nice.org.uk
O'Brien J, Ames D, Burns A (eds) Dementia, 2nd edn. Oxford: Arnold, 2000
Scott LJ, Goa KL. Galantamine. Drugs Aging 2000; 60:1095–122
Spencer CM, Noble S. Rivastigmine. Drugs Aging 1998; 13:391–411
Website: http://www.alzheimers.org.uk/news_events/m_facts.html

10 Clinical trial methodology

Introduction

■ A general definition of 'clinical trial', is any kind of study designed to establish the effects of a particular therapeutic intervention.
■ Table 10.1 gives some definitions of types of trials.

History

■ Clinical trials of some sort are probably as old as civilisation.
■ James Lind, an 18th-century Scottish physician is generally credited with having completed the first controlled trial – of vitamin C for scurvy.
■ Early Nobel prizes awarded in the field of psychiatry (Wagner-Jauregg in 1927 for 'malaria therapy' and Moniz in 1949 for the prefrontal leucotomy) have proven to be ineffective and abused respectively.
■ The gold standard of medical experimentation, the randomised control trial (RCT), was first used to evaluate the effects of antituberculous drugs in a trial sponsored by the Medical Research Council and published in 1948.
■ There is increasing interest in designing valid naturalistic or pragmatic trials to determine effectiveness in usual clinical practice.

Table 10.1 *Some commonly used terms to describe types of trials*

Term	Meaning
Controlled	A group receiving the investigative treatment is compared with another group receiving different treatment (e.g. placebo, no treatment or waiting list, another treatment of known efficacy). Usually applied to *prospective* (i.e. both groups are studied in parallel) rather than *retrospective* (i.e. using a historical control group treated at a previous time) trials
Placebo-controlled	One of the 'arms' of the trial is against a placebo condition. Usually required for a drug to be licensed
Randomised	Allocation to the different treatment 'arms' in the study is done randomly to minimise bias due to selection of patients for particular treatments
Open	Both clinician and patient know that a treatment is being given for a given indication. Open studies are usually uncontrolled (NB In clinical practice this is often equivalent to giving a therapeutic trial for an unlicensed indication)
Single-blind*	Usually taken to indicate that the assessing clinicians, but not the patients, are informed about which treatment is being given
Double-blind*	Neither the patient nor the assessing clinician are informed of which treatment is being given
Triple-blind*	Used when there are separate treating clinicians and assessors, both of whom, and the patient, are blind to treatment allocation
Naturalistic/pragmatic	Trials carried out in usual clinical practice with trade-off between rigorous trial methodology and 'real-world' applicability
Non-inferiority	Trials statistically powered to be able to detect a prespecified difference between two active drugs, which is judged to be clinically significant

*It is usually not checked/made clear whether blinding is successful in practice.

Drug development

■ New drugs can be developed by:
  – isolating the active ingredients in natural compounds;
  – modifying the chemistry of other drugs and;
  – from theoretical extension of basic science knowledge.

■ Only about one in every 10 000 potential products reach the market, often taking 10 years or more and many millions of pounds. Given the limited patent life (20 years in UK from the time of compound synthesis) drug companies often adopt aggressive marketing strategies to recoup their costs and deliver profits for shareholders.

■ A new drug is first tested in animals, to establish potential for desired effects and absence of unexpected or undesirable effects, before going through the four phases in humans (Table 10.2).

■ Phase I trials determine basic pharmacological parameters in human volunteers, e.g. pharmacokinetics, adverse effects, tolerance:
  – They are usually open or uncontrolled.
  – Adverse effects are often measured both subjectively and objectively (e.g. heart rate, blood pressure, neuropsychological, EEG, etc.).
  – Generally require 24-hour clinical observations and often exclude the young, women and the old because effects in humans are unknown; however, a drug safe in adult men, for example, may not be safe in children, women and the aged.
  – Because studies are uncontrolled some of the effects will be placebo effects.

■ Phase II trials establish whether or not a given drug works in a variety of conditions.
  – They are usually controlled, in that some patients get placebo.
  – In 'dose-ranging studies', to determine optimal dosage, each group of patients getting a particular dose of the drug can be thought of as a control group for the others.

■ Phase III, sometimes called 'comparative' trials, seek to determine the effects of a new drug with reference to those commonly used in clinical practice:
  – They are usually randomised with a proportion placebo controlled (a variety of other types of trial may be randomised and/or controlled but these are rarely used in drug development studies, see below).
  – They tend to be larger than Phase II studies.
  – Their major aim is to satisfy regulatory authorities and achieve a product licence.

■ Phase IV clinical 'trials' refer to the various methods of surveillance (see below) to establish the frequency of any serious or unexpected adverse effects of a drug once it has been licensed and introduced into regular clinical practice:
  – Similar to audit (measuring performance against a standard) and naturalistic outcome studies.

Table 10.2 *Phases of drug development*

	Question addressed	Main methods
Preclinical	Pharmacology and toxicology	Biochemical and animal studies
Phase I	Basic human pharmacology	Open/uncontrolled
Phase II	Efficacy in disease(s)	Controlled trials/small randomised controlled trials
Phase III	Efficacy and comparative efficacy (for regulatory approval)	Randomised controlled trials
Phase IV	Problems in clinical practice/ comparison with other drugs	Observational studies/randomised controlled trials

Designing or appraising a clinical trial (Table 10.3)

Table 10.3 *Questions relating to designing or appraising a clinical trial*

1. What is the aim or hypothesis of the study?
2. Which patients are to be studied?
3. What intervention is being studied?
4. What type of clinical trial is appropriate?
5. Was randomisation appropriately carried out?
6. Which outcomes should be measured and how?
7. Were appropriate statistical tests used?

What is the aim or hypothesis of the study?

Any study has a better chance of answering a single specific question rather than a number of less focused objectives. The question has to be:

■ clinically relevant (i.e. the answer will help make therapeutic decisions);
■ ethically acceptable (see below); and
■ not answered already (e.g. in a systematic review or meta-analysis), though replication of a finding in just one or two previous studies is reasonable.

Which patients are to be studied?

■ This is a matter of stipulating criteria for inclusion and exclusion.
■ Theoretical tension between recruiting a 'pure' highly selected group and an unselected heterogeneous group. The former reduces variance in the data and hence can produce more reliable results, but the findings may

not be representative of the entire patient population. The latter may be more valid but it may be difficult to identify a given effect.

■ In practice, broader inclusion criteria and minimal exclusions aid recruitment (particularly considering refusal and inability to give valid informed consent).

■ Many psychiatric studies exclude patients with comorbid substance abuse which comprise about half of all the patients seen clinically. This:
  – leaves uncertainty about efficacy in the comorbid group;
  – probably overestimates the benefits of any treatment in practice (noncompliance is high in comorbid patients).

■ The usual practice of excluding patients <16–18 and >60–65 years of age means that they often have to be treated without information from clinical trials, and usually 'off licence'.

■ Involuntarily detained patients cannot be enrolled in clinical trials for ethical reasons, resulting in the most severely ill patients often being treated in the absence of reliable evidence.

■ The trial setting determines the type of patients to whom the results will apply (inpatients, day patients, outpatients and/or those in primary care).

Which intervention is being studied?

■ Consider the type, formulation, dose, dosing schedule and route of administration of the medication.

■ Fixed versus flexible dosing:
  – results from fixed-dose trials generally easier to interpret but are different from how a drug is used in clinical practice and many patients will receive nonoptimal doses.
  – results from flexible dosing (tailoring the dose to a particular patient) are more clinically representative but can be difficult if the responsible clinician is blind to the treatment given.

■ What, if any, other drugs are permissible for participating patients, e.g. antipsychotic trials usually permit anticholinergic drugs and 'rescue' medication for behavioural disturbance.

■ Duration:
  – most trials are short (six weeks or less) simply because they are easier to do (Fig. 10.1)
  – long trials are complex, expensive and liable to have large numbers of people dropping out. Greater than a 20% drop-out may mean dubious representativeness and reliability (but hard to avoid in many psychiatric studies, especially long-term ones).

– ideally, clinical practice should be informed by long-term clinical trials, particularly if we advise our patients to stay on a drug for one year or more, but this needs to be balanced against the likelihood of higher drop-out rates.

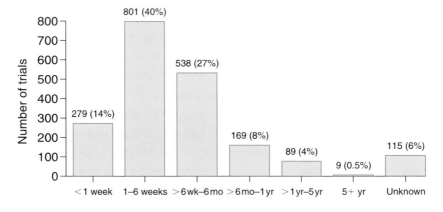

Figure 10.1 *Duration of the first 2000 clinical trials in schizophrenia.*
(Reproduced by permission from Thornley B, Adams C. BMJ 1998; 317:1181–4.)

What type of clinical trial is appropriate?

Randomised controlled trials (RCTs) were devised to measure drug efficacy and probably offer the greatest precision. However, they are not without problems and alternative approaches may be sufficient or optimum, depending on the specific clinical question. RCTs measure clinical *efficacy* (how well a drug works in ideal conditions). Pragmatic (or naturalistic) trials measure clinical *effectiveness* (how well a drug works in usual clinical practice).

Nonspecific effects

Studies are inescapably confounded by nonspecific effects which lead to improvement in the absence of any specific pharmacological action of the drug being studied:

■ Response rates on placebo can be very high (e.g. 30–40% in 8-week antidepressant studies).
■ Placebo response rates positively correlate with the year of study publication, i.e. rates are increasing. This may relate to increasing use of more mildly ill patients (see below).
■ These may lead to:
  – incorrect assumption of efficacy in uncontrolled trials; and

- incorrect assumption of inefficacy in underpowered studies due to type II statistical errors. Also
- Questioning of clinical significance even if statistical significance is attained as a high response rate to placebo tends to lead to smaller drug-effect sizes.

There are three main components to the nonspecific response:
- Measurement effects:
  - Whenever a population is chosen for an extreme characteristic above a specific cut-off (e.g. psychiatric rating score > x) then a second measurement will tend to be less extreme simply because of less-than-perfect reliability in repeated measurement (called *regression to the mean*).
  - Observer expectation: rating values may be elevated to include patients in a trial; subsequent ratings may be more objective or subject to expectation of improvement over time.
- Placebo effects (genuine but nonspecific treatment effects):
  - In RCTs, patients assigned to the placebo arm receive regular visits to their doctor and supportive help. This constitutes a treatment in its own right.
  - Patient (and doctor) expectations may recruit a nonpharmacological healing process. This factor may be greater in more mildly ill patients and those with greater self-motivation recruited from advertisements.
- Spontaneous recovery. This is difficult to distinguish from a placebo effect and reflects the natural history of the disorder. It is likely to be greater in more mildly ill patients with shorter length of illness.

Types of trials
- Uncontrolled trials:
  - can establish whether a treatment works at all and the profile of adverse effects;
  - however, nonspecific/placebo effects cannot be excluded in the absence of a control group.
- Controlled trials:
  - allow evaluation against placebo or a pre-existing treatment;
  - may reduce or control for placebo effects;
  - in the absence of randomisation are still subject to selection bias (conscious or unconscious). Patients getting a new treatment tend to be less severely ill and/or have better prognosis. Beneficial effects of new drugs are typically overestimated by 30–40%.

- RCTs:
  - randomisation increases the scientific quality or 'internal validity' of a trial (see below);
  - there are problems with 'external validity', i.e. patients able to give informed consent and willing to be randomised tend to differ from many potential participants. This limits their representativeness and hence the generalisability of the results to all patients;
  - RCTs designed to show a greater effect than placebo (with sufficient statistical power) are required to establish efficacy. RCTs against comparator drugs are frequently too poorly powered to be able to show a difference, and claims of equal efficacy need to be treated with caution. Recently so called *noninferiority* studies have been used in this situation. These are designed to have sufficient statistical power to detect a predefined difference between drugs, which is believed to be of clinical importance (see 'Power calculation' p. 155).
- Pragmatic trials:
  - Have more external but less internal validity.
  - Patient groups are representative, the interventions are routinely feasible and outcome measures are clinically relevant.
  - One option is to enrol patients for whom the clinician is uncertain as to which treatment should be prescribed.
  - Pragmatic trials are increasingly being applied in psychiatry.
- Patient preference trials:
  - Are a specific type of pragmatic trial.
  - Patients not willing to be randomised are given their preferred treatment. They are followed-up as in the trial and their results are compared with those who were randomised.
- Crossover trials:
  - All participants receive two (or more) interventions one after the other, with the two groups receiving a different treatment first.
  - Useful in relatively rare diseases where small numbers do not permit an RCT.
  - However, it is difficult to ensure that the trial is long enough to see therapeutic effects but short enough to avoid natural fluctuations confounding the trial.
  - Also there is the problem of carry-over effects from first treatment period to the second, and the potential for drug interactions.
  - 'Wash-out periods' of no treatment introduce new difficulties with sudden cessation of potentially effective treatments.

- N-of-1 trials:
  - Are crossover trials in which a patient is given two treatments. May be useful if it is not known which treatment they may benefit from.
  - Require patient consent and co-operation from the hospital pharmacy.
- Audit and naturalistic outcome studies:
  - Not usually thought of as clinical trials but are similar to Phase IV 'trials'.
  - Are uncontrolled and therefore unreliable even if patients are used as their own 'historical control'.
  - Nevertheless may provide valuable effectiveness information.

Was randomisation appropriately carried out?

- Two main purposes of randomisation:
  - To evenly distribute known and unknown confounders (e.g. age, sex, prognostic factors) affecting outcome.
  - To avoid selection bias (depends on concealing allocation).
- Successful randomisation is inversely related to the chance of a trial finding a treatment effect (in one review, 58% of randomised studies, where allocation could have been compromised, found a benefit of the new treatment versus 9% of randomised trials with adequate allocation concealment).
- Note that allocation concealment in randomisation is different to blinding (see Table 10.1).
- Allocation concealment:
  - requires unpredictable randomisation schedule, i.e. not dates of birth, day of week, etc.;
  - otherwise investigators may subvert randomisation.
- Ideally randomisation consists of:
  - assignment by random numbers (tossing a coin acceptable);
  - treatment assignment only revealed after consent to participate obtained (preferably by independent person);
  - methods include sealed opaque envelopes, telephoning centralised allocation unit.
- Randomisation methods to ensure that trial groups are balanced in terms of number and/or patient characteristics:
  - *'Blocked'* in groups (of four, six, etc.) to ensure broadly equal numbers in groups.
  - *'Stratified'* to ensure possible prognostic factors (e.g. age, sex, duration of illness, etc.) are balanced – requires randomisation schedule for each stratum.

- *'Minimisation'* in which subsequent patients are allocated by minimising differences in important variables.

■ Cluster trials are those in which subjects are randomised in groups or clusters – most common for wider aspects of health services than one particular treatment, e.g. effects of education on general practitioners done by group practice. The main disadvantage is that the unit of randomisation should be the unit of analysis requiring large numbers of individuals for adequate power.

Which outcomes should be measured and how?

■ Clinical outcomes can be measured either categorically (e.g. recovered/not recovered) or continuously (e.g. symptom severity scales).
■ Categorical outcomes:
  - are easiest to understand and are potentially the most clinically meaningful;
  - but may be determined from arbitrary cut-off points on rating scales or other measures (e.g. response measured as a percentage reduction in symptom severity);
  - requires nonparametric statistics.
■ Outcomes:
  - Should be prespecified (typically symptom severity scores) but might include adverse effects, drop-outs, quality-of-life measures, etc.
  - Multiple outcome measures increase finding statistically significant differences by chance.
■ Ratings scales:
  - If observer-rated scales are used, these should be reliable (when rated by two or more observers) and should be sensitive to change.
  - Psychiatry has had a surfeit of rating scales making comparison between trials problematic.
  - Researchers who use self-devised scales are more likely to report statistically significant effects than if they use standard measures.
■ Blinding:
  - Aim is to reduce bias and placebo effects (see Table 10.1).
  - Is rarely entirely successful (response or side-effects may reveal which treatment has been given).
  - Independent outcome assessors may mitigate these problems to some degree.

- Success of blinding can be checked by asking participants/assessors which treatment they believed they received.

Were appropriate statistical tests used?

■ Effect size and significance:
  - Care should be taken to distinguish between statistical and clinical significance.
  - Clinical significance relates to the magnitude of the effect size (e.g. is the advantage of the drug over placebo big enough to be clinically relevant?).
  - The effect size needed to reach clinical significance is arbitrarily determined.
  - The smaller the effect size the larger the sample needed to have a chance of detecting a statistically significant effect (see 'Power calculation' below). Beware of large samples with statistically significant but clinically irrelevant findings. (NB On its own, the size of the P value is not an indicator of the effect size or clinical significance.)
■ Power calculation:
  - This is necessary to determine the number of participants needed to detect a given finding at a specified level of statistical significance. This requires a defined primary outcome measure with estimation of numbers achieving a categorical outcome or likely mean difference continuous measure with its likely variance.
  - It is standard to aim for 90% power to detect a given effect size with $P < 0.05$ difference but different values can be specified. Various methods are available to calculate this, e.g. tables, computerised statistical packages.
■ Size of trial:
  - Most early RCTs in depression or schizophrenia had less than 60 participants (see Fig. 10.2). This is just about adequate to identify significant differences between an active treatment and placebo, depending on the effect size.
  - Trials comparing two active agents require much larger groups as the difference is generally much smaller.
  - Larger trials more accurately measure outcomes because the patients are likely to be more representative, measurement error is reduced and they tend to be better planned and organised.
  - Very large (mega) trials, including thousands of patients, are the best way of asking important therapeutic questions but there is a risk that small, clinically insignificant differences will be found.

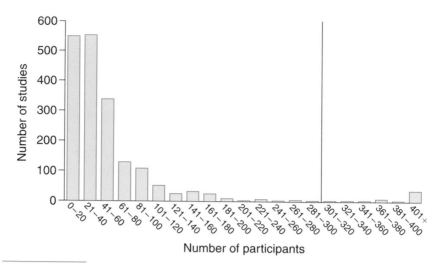

Figure 10.2 *The size of the first 2000 controlled trials in schizophrenia.* Line indicates number of patients required to find a 20% difference between treatments with standard power. (Reproduced with permission from Thornley B, Adams C. BMJ 1998; 317:1181–4.)

■ Types of analysis:
  – Particular statistical tests used depend on the properties of the data.
  – Continuous measures provide more statistical power than categorical ones. The latter has advantages when dealing with drop-outs from the trial before completion.
  – In intention-to-treat (ITT) analysis all randomised participants are included, i.e. including treatment drop-outs. With categorical measures, drop-outs are usually assigned to the poor outcome group. May under- or overestimate efficacy, and difficult to interpret if high rate of drop-outs or if the rate differs between treatments.
  – Last observation carried forward (LOCF) analysis is the standard approach with a continuous measure using the last available measure as the final measure. This may be ITT if includes baseline data or may only include subjects who have completed a certain period of treatment (e.g. two weeks). May over- or underestimate efficacy (Fig. 10.3).
  – Recently it has been suggested that a likelihood-based mixed effects model repeated measures (MMRM) approach gives a better estimate of outcome than the traditional LOCF approach. This models the time-course for missing data rather than carrying forward the last value unchanged. It may be more robust than LOCF and avoids both under- and overestimates of treatment effect with the latter.
  – Completer analysis includes only those who are still in the trial at the end. Overestimates treatment effects and is generally to be avoided.

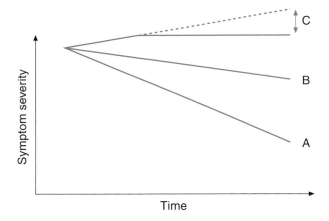

Figure 10.3 *The responses of three hypothetical participants in a trial. Patient A has a good response, B a minimal improvement and C drops out as condition is deteriorating. In this case, in a LOCF analysis, overall symptom deterioration will be underestimated by the size of the arrow and the treatment will appear better, especially with large numbers of drop-outs. However, depending on the disorder, the opposite is possible; if drop-outs are due to improvement or incidental factors then these patients may also improve and sometimes those deteriorating/improving after drop-out will be equal. The point is, we just don't know what happened to these people.*

■ Problematic analyses:
 – The success of randomisation should not be tested by comparing descriptive variables; some will differ by chance.
 – Defining subgroups of patients by who responded particularly well or badly to treatment and taking this to indicate that certain groups should get particular treatments. The exception is if there was a prespecified hypothesis. Subgroup analysis is acceptable if clearly presented as exploratory, i.e. for future hypothesis testing.
 – Multiple hypothesis testing. One statistical comparison in 20 is likely to be significant at $P < 0.05$ by chance alone. It is acceptable if there are prespecified hypotheses but correction for multiple testing should be made. Exploratory testing ('data dredging') is acceptable if clearly stated as such.
■ Meta-analysis:
 – Individual RCTs and pragmatic primary research studies are prone to bias, random variation and type II errors. Meta-analysis is a method of pooling results from individual studies to increase power.
 – They must be part of a systematic review to attempt to get all relevant studies to avoid selection bias; nevertheless, publication bias is possible as negative RCTs may be unpublished.

- The methods of study selection, data extraction and subsequent combination can vary tremendously and can greatly influence the conclusions drawn.
- Evidence-based medicine projects such as the Cochrane Collaboration aim to improve the registration of clinical trials and the synthesis of results (http://www.cochrane.org).

Ethical considerations

■ Ethical issues apply to all stages of any trial – The Declaration of Helsinki (fifth revision) applies (see http://www.wma.net/e/policy/b3.htm).

■ Planning a trial:
- The trial should address an unresolved question.
- With methods likely to provide a useful answer, e.g. be sufficiently powered.
- A recent issue has been the ethics of placebo control in conditions such as schizophrenia and depression where standard treatments are effective.
- Attention needs to be paid to what treatment is offered at the termination of the trial, particularly if patients have been treated with placebo.
- Ethical approval is required with patient information and consent forming an important aspect of the application.
- Drugs unlicensed for a particular indication need specific trial approval from the regulatory authorities (Medicines and Healthcare products Regulatory Authority in the UK) with new regulations implementing the European Union Directive 2001/20/EC on Good Clinical Practice in Clinical Trials coming into force in May 2004 (see http://www.mhra.gov.uk)

■ Consent:
- Fully informed, usually written, consent is required – participants should fully appreciate the nature of the trial and the potential risks and benefits.
- May be a particular problem in psychiatry with recent concerns about consent even in relatively stable psychotic patients – this appears related to cognitive impairment and can be dealt with by appropriate education.
- Third party consent may be appropriate good practice if a participant cannot consent but lacks legal force and is likely to reduce enrolment.

■ Conduct of trial:
- Good clinical practice guidelines apply, e.g Association of British Pharmaceutical Industry Guidelines and EU Directives.

- Payment or inducement are not allowed but compensation can be given, e.g. for travel and subsistence. Healthy volunteers can also receive compensation for inconvenience or discomfort.
- Insurance or indemnity agreement may be necessary for adverse effects.
- Research data are confidential and should be stored anonymously and safely.
■ Fraudulent analysis or presentation of results of a trial is unethical and may be misleading or dangerous.

Postmarketing surveillance/Phase IV clinical trials

Some important adverse effects detected by postmarketing surveillance are shown in Table 10.4.

Table 10.4 *Some important adverse effects detected by postmarketing surveillance*

Year	Drug	Adverse effect
1961	Thalidomide	Phocomelia**
1963	MAOIs	Cheese reactions
1976	Clozapine	Agranulocytosis*
1979–90	Mianserin	Blood dyscrasia*
1983	Zimelidine	Hypersensitivity reactions and Guillain–Barré syndrome**
1986	Nomifensine	Haemolytic anaemia**
1990	Pimozide	Ventricular arrhythmias*
1993	Remoxipride	Aplastic anaemia**
1999	Vigabatrin	Visual field defects*
1999	Sertindole	Sudden (cardiac) death**
2001	Droperidol	QT prolongation on ECG**
2001	Thioridazine	QT prolongation on ECG*
2003	Nefazodone	Hepatotoxicity** (*in US)

* Leading to requirements for appropriate monitoring (and usually restricted use).
** Leading to product withdrawal (or highly restricted use).

Voluntary reporting
■ Depends upon the observational skills and conscientiousness of individual clinicians.
■ Countries have national reporting systems. In the UK the Committee for the Safety of Medicines/Medicine and Healthcare products Regulatory Agency (http://www.mca.gov.uk) encourage notification of possible

adverse reactions for new products (indicated by 'black triangles') using a 'yellow cards' reporting system.

■ National centres can send such information to the WHO Collaborating Centre for International Drug Monitoring.

■ The method:
  - is cheap;
  - probably underestimates serious adverse effects and is inadequate as an epidemiological tool;
  - has identified adverse effects resulting in withdrawal of particular products, e.g. remoxipride.

Intensive surveillance

■ More intensive surveillance is expensive and usually restricted to hospital inpatients.

■ Examples include the Boston Collaborative Drug Surveillance Programme (http://www.bu.edu/bcdsp) and the Medicines Evaluation and Monitoring Group (MEMO) in the UK.

Retrospective studies

■ These are more expensive but much more informative than simple voluntary systems.

■ Drawbacks are those of selection bias and unavailablity of information

■ Examples include:
  - simple case-control studies;
  - the Retrospective Assessment of Drug Safety (RADS) programme;
  - pre-existing data storage systems, such as the Office of Population Censuses and Surveys (OPCS) data;
  - the UK-based General Practice Research Database, e.g. recently reported an increased risk of venous thromboembolism on antipsychotic drugs.

■ Databases can be linked by computer, e.g. people exposed to a particular product, and people admitted to hospital with a particular problem. Linking a national registry of clozapine recipients to national death records found that clozapine increased the risk of fatal pulmonary embolism and respiratory disorders but reduced the risk of suicide.

Prospective studies

■ These are the most reliable but also the most expensive.

■ Examples are:
- A new product may be released with recorded/registered prescriptions to facilitate monitoring.
- An established product can be monitored, e.g. prompted blood tests with clozapine.
- Prescription event monitoring (PEM). A standard cohort study of the first 10 000 patients exposed to a particular drug. This is sufficiently powerful to detect an adverse reaction risk of 0.1% but relies on accurate reporting and has been known to miss important adverse effects.

Conclusions

■ Patients need protection from unscrupulous or overenthusiastic triallists, but trials are needed to establish effective new treatments.

■ The 'explanatory' RCT has given clinical therapeutics a sound scientific base but measures efficacy rather than effectiveness.

■ Pragmatic clinical trials and multicentre studies in psychiatry are in their infancy but have much to commend them in determining effectiveness in clinical practice.

■ Single trials can be cited to prove virtually anything and results need independent replication.

■ Systematic reviews and meta-analyses can reliably synthesise available evidence but are no better than the studies they contain.

■ Psychiatrists have been overreliant on the pharmaceutical industry to evaluate new products and have failed to date to conduct any independent large/mega trials.

References

Key references
Carpenter WT Jr, Gold JM, Lahti AC *et al*. Decisional capacity for informed consent in schizophrenia research. Arch Gen Psychiatry 2000; 57:533–8.
Chalmers TC, Celano P, Sacks HS, Smith H Jr. Bias in treatment assignment in controlled clinical trials. N Engl J Med 1983; 309:1358–61
Even C, Siobud-Dorocant E, Dardennes RM. Critical approach to antidepressant trials. Blindness protection is necessary, feasible and measurable. Br J Psychiatry 2000; 177:47–51
Moncrieff J, Wessely S, Hardy R. Meta-analysis of trials comparing antidepressants with active placebos. Br J Psychiatry 1998; 172:227–31; discussion 232–4

Schulz KF, Chalmers I, Hayes RJ, Altman DG. Empirical evidence of bias. Dimensions of methodological quality associated with estimates of treatment effects in controlled trials. JAMA 1995; 273:408–12

Thornley B, Adams C. Content and quality of 2000 controlled trials in schizophrenia over 50 years. BMJ 1998; 317:1181–4

Vastag B. Helsinki discord? A controversial declaration. JAMA 2000; 284:2983–85

Walker AM, Lanza LL, Arellano F, Rothman KJ. Mortality in current and former users of clozapine. Epidemiology 1997; 8:671–7

Zornberg GL, Jick H. Antipsychotic drug use and risk of first-time idiopathic venous thromboembolism: a case-control study. Lancet 2000; 356:1219–23

Further reading

Bedi N, Chilvers C, Churchill R *et al*. Assessing effectiveness of treatment of depression in primary care. Partially randomised preference trial. Br J Psychiatry 2000; 177:312–18

Edwards IR, Aronson JK. Adverse drug reactions: definitions, diagnosis, and management. Lancet 2000; 356:1255–9

Guyatt G, Sackett D, Taylor DW *et al*. Determining optimal therapy – randomized trials in individual patients. N Engl J Med 1986; 314:889–92

Hotopf M, Churchill R, Lewis G. Pragmatic randomised controlled trials in psychiatry. Br J Psychiatry 1999; 175:217–23

Kunz R, Oxman AD. The unpredictability paradox: review of empirical comparisons of randomised and non-randomised clinical trials. BMJ 1998; 317:1185–90

Lawrie SM, McIntosh AM, Rao S. Critical Appraisal for Psychiatry. Edinburgh: Churchill Livingstone, 2000

Louis TA, Lavori PW, Bailar JCD, Polansky M. Crossover and self-controlled designs in clinical research. N Engl J Med 1984; 310:24–31

Marshall M, Lockwood A, Bradley C *et al*. Unpublished rating scales: a major source of bias in randomised controlled trials of treatments for schizophrenia. Br J Psychiatry 2000; 176:249–52

Pocock SJ. Clinical Trials: A Practical Approach. Chichester: John Wiley, 1983

Savulescu J, Chalmers I, Blunt J. Are research ethics committees behaving unethically? Some suggestions for improving performance and accountability. BMJ 1996; 313:1390–3

Index

Page numbers in *italics* refer to tables and figures.

Abbreviated Mental Test Score (AMTS) 139
absorption of drugs *29*, *29*, *30*
acamprosate 115
acetylcholine (ACh)
    pathways in the brain 20
    receptors 22–3
    synthesis and metabolism *13*, 20, *137*
acetylcholinesterase 20, *22*, *137*
activities of daily living (ADL) 139
acute dystonia 47, *47*
acute mania, efficacy of lithium 82
Adam 120
Adderall XR® 128
adenosine monophosphate (AMP) 7, *8*,
    12, *16*, *21*, 117
adenosine triphosphate (ATP) *8*
adenylate cyclase *7*, *9*
ADHD *see* attention deficit/hyperactivity
    disorder
administration of drugs *30*
adolescent psychopharmacology 123–34
β-adrenoceptor antagonists 106
adrenoceptors 16
agonists 37, *37*
akathisia 48
alcohol
    comorbidity 115–16
    history 109
    neuropharmacology 111–13, *114*
    treatment of dependence 114–15
    withdrawal 113, *113*
allocation concealment 153
alprazolam *102*

Alzheimer's disease
    cholinergic hypothesis 137, *137*
    drug intervention targets *22*, 23,
        136–7
    mechanism of neuronal damage 138
    monoamine deficits 138
    pathology *136*
    risk factors *136*
Alzheimer's Disease Assessment Scale 138
amfebutamone (bupropion) 120
amfetamine *14*, *17*, 18, 119
γ-aminobutyric acid *see* GABA
    (γ–aminobutyric acid)
amisulpride 53
amnesia, after ECT 77
AMPA (amino-3-hydroxy-5-methyl-4-
    isoxazole proprionate) 9, 24, 115
amygdala 96
amyloid precursor protein (APP) *136*
amytriptyline *64*
anandamide 6
antagonists 38–9, *38*, *39*
anticholinesterase inhibitors 135,
    139–42
anticonvulsant drugs 87–92
    see also electroconvulsive therapy
        (ECT)
antidepressant drugs
    anxiety 105–6
    autism 130
    bipolar disorder 92–3
    choice of 72
    comorbid depression and alcohol
        abuse 115–16

antidepressant drugs (contd)
dementia 143
depression in children and
adolescents 131–2
effective use 72
history 59
neurotrophic/neuroplastic
hypotheses 62–3
pharmacology *64*
serotonin (5-HT) hypothesis 60, *60*
treatment resistance 72–3
types *see specific drug types*
see also depression; electroconvulsive
therapy (ECT)
antipsychotic drugs 41–58
adverse effects 47–51, *47, 49, 51*
anxiety 107
atypical *see* atypical antipsychotic
drugs
autism 130–1
bipolar disorder 92
chemical classification *45*
dementia 143–4
dopamine hypothesis 41–4, *42, 43, 44*
and dopamine receptor subtypes 44–5
history 41
indications *45*
therapeutic actions 46–7
anxiety
children and adolescents 133
comorbid alcohol abuse 116
neurobiology 96
neurochemistry 96–8
anxiolytic drugs 95–108
AP5 (2-amino-5-phosphopentanoic acid)
25
apomorphine 14
area under the curve (AUC) 28, *29*
aripiprazole 53–4
aspirin 142
atomoxetine 129
attention deficit/hyperactivity disorder
(ADHD)
clinical background 123–4
non-pharmacological treatments 125
pharmacological treatments 125–9
scientific background 124
atypical antipsychotic drugs
atypicality defined 51
autism 131
bipolar disorder 92
chemical classification *45*
distribution of pharmacological
mechanisms 52–3
dopamine receptor affinities 44

drugs 53–7
history 41
mechanisms of atypicality 52
atypical depression 69, 105
audit 153
autism
features 129–30
pharmacological treatments 130–1
autoreceptors 10–11, *10*

barbiturates 23
BDZs *see* benzodiazepines (BDZs)
behavioural and psychiatric symptoms
of dementia (BPSD) 135, 143–4
behavioural therapy, ADHD 125
benzhexol (trihexphenidyl) 48
benzodiazepines (BDZs) 98–104
actions *100*
adverse effects *101*
clinical efficacy 100–1, 113, 133
GABA$_A$–BZD receptor complex 23,
24, 98–100, *99*
history of prescription 95, *95*
paediatric anxiety 133
pharmacokinetics 101–2, *101, 102*
place in clinical practice 104
in pregnancy 104
prescription guidelines 104
tolerance 102–3
toxicity in overdose 104
withdrawal syndrome 103, *103*
benztropine 14
beta blockers (β-adrenoceptor
antagonists) 106
bicuculline *24*
bioavailability 27
bipolar disorder
children and adolescents 132
drug management 79–94
blinding *146*, 154–5
blood–brain barrier *31*, 32
brain aversion system 96
brain-derived neurotrophic factor 6
bromocriptine 50
buprenorphine *117*, 118
bupropion (amfebutamone) 120
buspirone 104–5, 116
butyrophenones 41
butyrylcholinesterase 137

calcium (Ca^{2+}) channel antagonists
(blockers) 33, 90
cannabinoid receptors 6
cannabis 110, 121
carbamazepine 89–90, 113

carbon dioxide (CO$_2$) and panic   97–8
catechol-O-methyltransferase (COMT)
    14, 17
cation transport, effects of lithium   80
β-CCE (ethyl-β-carboline-3-carboxylate)
    99
child and adolescent
    psychopharmacology   123–34
chlorpromazine   41, 46
cholecystokinin (CCK)   4, 5, 98
cholinergic neurones, sites of drug
    action   *22*
cholinergic neurotransmission, effects of
    lithium   80–1
cholinergic precursors   139
cholinergic receptors   22–3
cholinesterase inhibitors   135, 139–42
citalopram   *66*
Clinical Dementia Rating (CDR)   139
clinical trials   145–62
    defined   145
    design/appraisal *see* design/appraisal
        of clinical trials
    history   145
    postmarketing surveillance *see* post-
        marketing surveillance (phase IV
        trials)
    types   *146*
Clinical Trials Directive (EU)   158
Clinicians Interview Based Impression of
    Change (CIBIC)   139
clomipramine   *64*, 105, 106, 130
clonazepam   *99*
clonidine   *17*, 96
clozapine   41, 49, 52
cluster trials   154
C$_{max}$ (maximum plasma concentration)
    28, *29*
cocaine   118–19
Cochrane Collaboration   158
cognitive behavioural therapy (CBT)
    131, 133
cognitive impairment after ECT   77
comparative trials   147
completer analysis   156
consent   158
controlled drugs   110–11
controlled trials   *146*, 151
    see also randomised controlled trials
        (RCTs)
corticotrophin-releasing factor (CRF)
    receptors   5
cortisol   62
crack cocaine   118
crossover trials   152–3

cyclic adenosine monophosphate (cyclic
    AMP; cAMP)   7, *8*, 12, 16, *21*, 117
cytochrome P450 (CYP450) enzymes   33

dantroline   50
dementia, drug treatment   135–44
    Alzheimer's disease *see* Alzheimer's
        disease
    behavioural and psychiatric
        symptoms   135, 143–4
    dementia with Lewy bodies   138
    drug classes   139–43
    history   135
    outcome assessment   138–9
    vascular dementia   138
depression
    atypical   69, 105
    children and adolescents   131–2
    comorbid alcohol abuse   115–16
    dopamine in   61
    HPAA regulation abnormalities in   62
    lithium prophylaxis   83
    monoamine hypothesis   59–60, *60*
    noradrenaline in   61
    serotonin in   61
    treatment-resistant   72–3
    see also antidepressant drugs;
        electroconvulsive therapy (ECT)
design/appraisal of clinical trials
    aim/hypothesis   148
    duration   149–50, *150*
    ethical considerations   158–9
    interventions   149
    nonspecific effects   150–1
    outcome measurement   154–5
    patient recruitment   148–9
    randomisation   153–4
    statistical tests   155–8, *156, 157*
    trial size   155, *156*
    type of trial   150, 151–3
desipramine   128
dexamfetamine
    efficacy in ADHD   126
    guidance for use in ADHD   127–8
    interactions   *126*
    mechanism of action   125
    prescription for ADHD   127
    side effects   126
diazepam   95, *99, 101, 102*
dihydroxyphenylacetic acid (DOPAC)   14
disinhibition of neurones   *3*
distribution of drugs   *29*, 31–2, *31*
disulfiram   16, 114–15, *114*
dizocilpine (MK-801)   25
donepezil   141

dopamine agonists   48
dopamine (DA)
    amphetamine-induced release in
        schizophrenia   43, *43*
    in antipsychotic drug action   13, *14*,
        41–5, *42*, *43*, *44*
    and drugs of abuse   111, 112
    in major depression   61
    pathways in the brain   11–12, *11*
    receptors   12–13, *15*, 41–5, *42*, *44*
    synthesis and metabolism   12, *13*
dopaminergic neurones, sites of drug
    action   *14*
dosulepin (dothiepin)   *64*
drug administration routes   *30*
drug development   146–7, *148*
drugs of abuse
    and dopamine   111
    history   109–10
    legal issues (UK)   110–11
    reasons for use   109
    see also specific drugs
duloxetine   70
dyskinesia, tardive   48–9, *49*

Ecstasy   120
effect size   155
electroconvulsive stimulation (ECS)   62
electroconvulsive therapy (ECT)
    clinical uses   76
    contraindications   77
    effects on neurones   *63*
    efficacy   76
    history   74
    indications   74–5
    mode of action   74
    procedure   75
    side-effects   76–7
elimination of drugs   *29*, 32–5, *32*, *34*
enactogens   120
ergot derivatives   143
escitalopram   *66*, 67
ethanol *see* alcohol
ethics in clinical trials   158 9
ethyl-β-carboline-3-carboxylate (β-CCE)
    99
Eve   120
excretion of drugs   34
extrapyramidal side-effects (EPSE),
    antipsychotic drugs   47–9, *47*, *49*, 52

fenfluramine   *19*
first-order kinetics   27, *28*
first-pass effect   *30*
flumazenil   97, *99*, 100

fluoxetine   *66*, 132
flupentixol   42, *42*
fluphenazine   46
flurazepam   *102*
fluvoxamine   *66*, 130, 132, 133

GABA$_A$–BZD receptor complex   23, *24*,
    98–100, *99*
GABA (γ-aminobutyric acid)
    in anxiety   97
    effects of alcohol   112
    receptors   23–4, *24*
    synthesis and metabolism   13, 23
gabapentin   91
galantamine   141–2
generalised anxiety disorder (GAD)
    comorbid alcohol abuse   116
    drug treatment   101, 105, 106, 107,
        133
    NICE treatment guidelines   98
    serotonin in   97
genetics
    ADHD   124
    alcoholism   112
    Alzheimer's disease   *136*
    schizophrenia   42
Ginkgo biloba   143
glutamate
    current interest in   24–5
    effects of alcohol   112
    receptors   24–5, *25*
    synthesis and metabolism   *13*
G-protein receptors   7–8, *8*, *9*

half-life (t$_{1/2}$)   28, *29*
hallucinogens   110, 119
haloperidol
    autism treatment   130–1
    history   41
heroin   *117*
hormone replacement therapy (HRT)   142
HPA (hypothalmic–pituitary–adrenal)
    axis   62
5-HT$_{1A}$ receptor agonists   104–5
γ-hydroxybutyrate   *14*
5-hydroxyindoleacetic acid (5-HIAA)
    19, 120
5-hydroxytryptamine (5-HT) *see*
    serotonin (5-HT)
hyerkinetic disorder   123
hypnotic drugs, benzodiazepines   95,
    100, 102
hypocretins   5–6
hypothalmic–pituitary–adrenal (HPA)
    axis   62

imipramine 59, *64*, 105, 106, 129
Instrumental Activities of Daily Living
    (IADL) 139
intention-to-treat (ITT) analysis 156
interpersonal therapy (IPT) 131
Interview for Deterioration in Daily
    Living in Dementia (IDDD) 139
ion channels 7
ionotropic receptors 7, 25, *25*
iproniazid 59

kava kava 107
ketamine 25, 119
kindling 87

LAAM (levo-alpha-acetylmethadol) 118
lactation, use of lithium 85
lamotrigine 71, 90–1
last observation carried forward (LOCF)
    analysis 156, *157*
law of mass action 27, 37
levetiracetam 92
levo-alpha-acetylmethadol (LAAM) 118
lithium
    dosage 84
    drug interactions *86*
    history 79–80
    indications 82–3, 87
    initiation of therapy 84
    mode of action 80–1
    mortality of treated patients 87
    pharmacokinetics 81–2
    pregnancy and lactation 85
    renal function effects 85–6
    response predictors *83*
    side-effects 85
    toxicity 86
    treatment monitoring 84–5
    treatment-resistant depression 73
locus coeruleus 16
lofepramine *64*
lorazepam *102*
lysergic acid diethylamide (LSD) 110,
    119

Manchester and Oxford Universities
    Scale for the Psychopathological
    Assessment of Dementia
    (MOUSEPAD) 139
mania
    children and adolescents 132
    see also bipolar disorder
manic-depressive psychosis see bipolar
    disorder
MAOIs see monoamine oxidase

inhibitors (MAOIs)
marijuana (cannabis) 110, 121
measurement effects in clinical trials 151
memantine 135, 142
meta-analysis 157–8
metabolism of drugs 32–3
metabotropic receptors 7, 25
methadone *117*, 118
methylenedioxyamfetamine (MDA;
    Adam) 120
methylenedioxyethylamfetamine
    (MDEA; Eve) 120
methylenedioxymethamfetamine
    (MDMA; ecstasy) 120
methylphenidate
    efficacy in ADHD 126
    guidance for use in ADHD 127–8
    interactions *126*
    mechanism of action 125
    prescription for ADHD 127
    side-effects 126
α-methyltyrosine *17*
metrifonate 141
mianserin 71
mifepristone 62
milnacipran 70
Mini-Mental State Examination (MMSE)
    139
mirtazapine 71
Misuse of Drugs Act 1971 110–11
mixed effects model repeated measures
    (MMRM) 156
moclobemide 68, 69
monoamine hypothesis of depression
    59–60, *60*
monoamine oxidase inhibitors (MAOIs)
    contraindications 70
    efficacy 68–9, 105
    interactions 69
    neurochemistry 68
    pharmacokinetics 68
    side-effects 69
monoaminergic neurotransmission,
    effects of lithium 80
mood stabilisers 79–94
    defined 79
MOUSEPAD 139
Multimodal Treatment Study of ADHD
    128
muscarinic receptors 22–3
muscimol *24*

naltrexone 111, 115, 118
NARIs (noradrenaline re-uptake
    inhibitors) 70, 129

NaSSa (noradrenaline- and serotonin-specific antidepressant) 71
National Institute for Clinical Excellence (NICE) guidelines
  ADHD treatment 127
  Alzheimer's disease 135, 140, 142
  anxiety 98
  bipolar disorder treatment 93
  depression 72
  ECT 75
  prescription of cholinesterase inhibitors 140
  schizophrenia treatment 46
naturalistic outcome studies *146*, 153
nefazodone 70
neurokinins 4, *5*, 107
neuroleptic malignant syndrome (NMS) 50
neuromodulators 4, *5*
neurones, effects of stress and ECT *63*
neuropeptides 4, *5*, 113
neuropeptide Y (NPY) *5*, 113
neuroprotection, lithium 81
Neuropsychiatric Inventory (NPI) 139
neurosteroids 6
neurotensin 4, *5*
neurotransmission 1–26
  example of disinhibition *3*
  fast and slow 2, *2*
  process 1–3, *2*
neurotransmitters
  associated disorders *5*
  coexistent 3–4
  dysregulation in ADHD 124
  effects of drugs 35–6, *36*
  pathway organisation 6
  see also specific neurotransmitters
neurotransmitter receptors
  G-protein 7–8, *8*, *9*
  ion channel-linked 7
  locations 9–11, *10*
  types 7, *9*
NICE guidelines *see* National Institute for Clinical Excellence (NICE) guidelines
nicotine 120
nicotinic receptors 22
nimodipine 143
nitrazepam *102*
NMDA (*N*-methyl D-aspartate) receptors 25, *25*
n-of-1 trials 153
noninferiority studies *146*, 152
nonsteroidal anti-inflammatory drugs (NSAIDs) 136

nootropic drugs 142
noradrenaline (NA)
  in alcohol withdrawal 112
  in anxiety 96
  deficit in Alzheimer's disease 138
  in major depression 61
  pathways in the brain 16
  receptors (adrenoceptors) 16
  synthesis and metabolism *13*, 16
noradrenaline re-uptake inhibitors (NARIs) 70, 129
noradrenaline- and serotonin-specific antidepressant (NaSSa) 71
noradrenergic neurones, sites of drug action *17*
nortriptyline *64*

obsessive–compulsive disorder (OCD) 132–3
oestrogen 136
olanzapine 54, 71, 92, 131
opiates/opioids
  effects 116
  history 109–10
  substitute therapies 117–18, *117*
  terms 116
  withdrawal 117
orexins 5–6
outcome measurement in clinical trials 154–5
oxcarbazepine 90
oxiracetam 142

pallidotomy 49
panic attacks 4, 96, 97, 98, 116
panic disorder
  drug treatment 101, 105, 106, 107
  neurobiology 4, 96, 97, 98
  NICE treatment guidelines 98
parachloramfetamine *19*
parachlorophenylalanine *19*
pargyline *14*, *17*
Parkinson's disease 11, *22*
paroxetine *66*
patient preference trials 152
pemoline 128
pentoxyphylline 143
pentylenetetrazol 97
periaqueductal grey (PAG) 96
P-glycoprotein 32
pharmacodynamics 35–9
  agonists 37, *37*
  antagonists 38–9, *38*, *39*
  drug action on neurotransmitters 35–6, *36*

sensitisation 39, 111
tolerance 39
pharmacokinetics 27–35
  absorption *29, 29, 30*
  basic principles 27–9, *28, 29*
  distribution *29*, 31–2, *31*
  drug administration routes compared
    30
  elimination *29*, 32–5, *32, 34*
  see also specific drugs
phase I to IV clinical trials 147, *148*
  see also postmarketing surveillance
    (phase IV trials)
phencyclidine (PCP) 25, 119
phenelzine 14
phenolthiazines 41
phenotolamine *17*
phenoxybenzamine *17*
phenylpiperazines 70
phospholipid hydrolysis 8, *9*
piperoxane *17*
piracetam 142
placebo effects 151
postmarketing surveillance (phase IV
    trials)
  adverse effects detected *159*
  intensive 160
  prospective studies 161
  retrospective studies 160
  voluntary reporting 159–60
post-traumatic stress disorder (PTSD)
    96, 97, 106
potency 37
power calculation 155
pragmatic trials *146*, 152
pramiracetam 142
pregabalin 107
pregnancy
  complications with BDZs 104
  use of lithium 85
prescription event monitoring (PEM) 161
presynaptic heteroceptors 10, *10*
procyclidine 48
propentofylline 143
prospective studies 161
pseudo-parkinsonism 47, *47*
psychedelic drugs 110
PTSD (post-traumatic stress disorder)
    96, 97, 106
1-pyramidinyl piperazine (1-PP) 105

QTc, drug effects *45, 51*, 56, 57, 130
quetiapine 54–5, 131

randomisation 153–4
randomised controlled trials (RCTs)
    145, *146*, 152
ratings scales 154

reboxetine 70
regression to the mean 151
renal function, effects of lithium 85–6
reserpine *14, 17, 19*
retrospective studies 160
risperidone 55, 131
rivastigmine 141

St John's wort 71
salicylate 142
schizophrenia
  amphetamine-induced dopamine
    release 43, *43*
  comorbid substance abuse 116
  dopamine receptors in 44
  efficacy of α and β flupenthixol 42,
    42
  NICE treatment guidelines 46
  use of ECT 76
  see also antipsychotic drugs
second messenger systems
  effects of lithium 81
  G-protein receptor-linked 7–8, *8, 9*
sedation, antipsychotic drugs 46
selective serotonin re-uptake inhibitors
    (SSRIs)
  anxiety 106, 133
  autism 130
  comorbid depression and alcohol
    abuse 116
  comparative pharmacology *66*
  depression in children and
    adolescents 131–2
  discontinuation syndrome 68
  efficacy 66–7
  interactions 67
  neurochemistry 66
  obsessive–compulsive disorder 132–3
  pharmacokinetics 66
  serotonin syndrome 68
  side-effects 67
sensitisation 39, 111
serotonergic neurones, sites of drug
    action *19*
serotonin (5-HT)
  in alcoholism 112–13
  in anxiety 97
  deficit in Alzheimer's disease 138
  hypothesis of antidepressant drug
    action 60, *60*
  in major depression 61
  pathways 18
  receptors 19–20, *21*
  syndrome 68
  synthesis and metabolism *13*, 18–19
  see also 5-HT$_{1A}$ receptor agonists

serotonin and noradrenaline re-uptake
  inhibitors (SNRIs) 70
sertindole 55–6
sertraline *66*, 132, 133
significance (statistical) 155
sleep problems, use of benzodiazepines
  95, 100, 102
SNRIs (serotonin and noradrenaline
  re-uptake inhibitors) 70
sodium valproate 88–9
somatodendritic autoreceptors 10, *10*
SSRIs *see* selective serotonin re-uptake
  inhibitors (SSRIs)
statistical tests 155–8, *156*, *157*
steady-state concentration 35
stimulants
  ADHD treatment 125–8, *126*
  drugs of abuse 118–19
  history 110
  mode of action *14*, *17*, 125
stress, effects on neurones *63*
substance P 4, *5*, 107
substantia nigra 11
synaptic transmission 1–2, *2*
  see also neurotransmission

$t_{1/2}$ (half-life) 28, *29*
tacrine (tetrahydroaminoacridine; THA)
  135, 140–1
tardive syndromes *47*, 48–9, *49*
TCAs *see* tricyclic antidepressants
temazepam *102*
terminal autoreceptors 10, *10*
tetrabenazine *14*, *17*, *19*, 49
tetrahydroaminoacridine (tacrine; THA)
  135, 140–1
tetrahydrocannabinol (THC) *3*, 121
therapeutic index 35
thiamine deficiency in alcoholics 113
thyrotrophin-releasing hormone (TRH) 4
tiagabine 91–2
tobacco 110

tolerance 39
topiramate 91, 115
tranquillisation, antipsychotic drugs 46
trazodone 70
TRH (thyrotrophin-releasing hormone) 4
tricyclic antidepressants (TCAs)
  ADHD 128–9
  anxiety 105, 106, 133
  comparative pharmacology *64*
  contraindications 65
  depression in children and
    adolescents 131
  efficacy 65
  interactions 65
  neurochemistry 63
  pharmacokinetics 64
  side-effects 65
tropolone *14*
tryptophan 18, *19*, 71
tyrosine hydroxylase *14*, *17*

uncontrolled trials 151

valproate semisodium 88
valproate/valproic acid 88–9
vascular dementia 138, 142–3
velnacrine 140–1
venlafaxine 70, 105
ventral tegmental area (VTA) *3*, *11*
vitamin supplements 113, 136

yohimbine *17*, 96

zaleplon 99, *102*
zero-order kinetics 27, *28*
ziprasidone 56
zolpidem 99, *102*
zonisamide 92
zopiclone 23, 99, *102*
zotepine 56–7
zuclopenthixol *45*